Diagnosis Parkinson's Disease...Now What?

A Guide For Patients and Caregivers

Rory M. Graham

Diagnosis Parkinson's Disease...Now What? © 2023

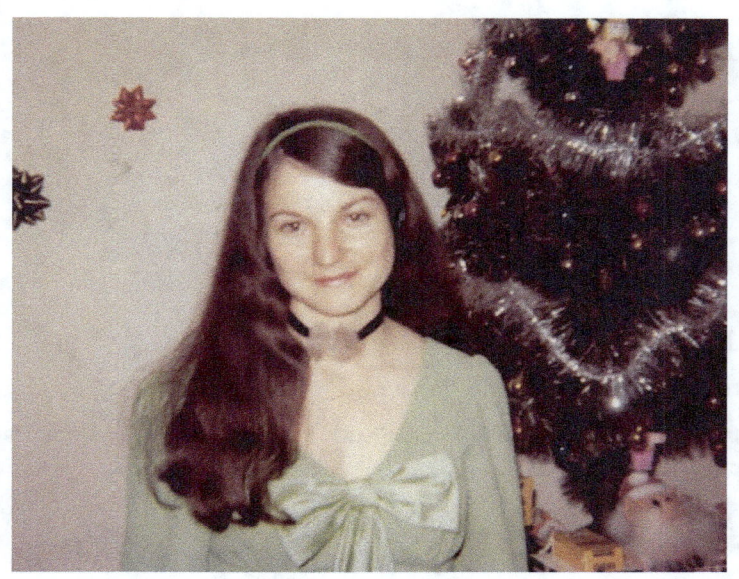

This book is dedicated to my soulmate
and the love of my life, Zelia Graham.

Table of Content

Introduction

Imagine facing a relentless opponent, an unseen adversary that targets the very core of your being. A silent attacker, shrouded in mystery, threatening to steal the vibrancy of life you once cherished. This isn't the plot of a thriller; it's the harsh reality for millions battling Parkinsonism—a world of neurodegenerative turmoil where the brain becomes the battleground, and abnormal proteins assume the role of the formidable antagonist. As of 2023, more than 10 million people have been diagnosed with Parkinson's Disease. The lives of those diagnosed and their loved ones ground to a halt as they face the harrowing journey of managing a condition that has no known cure.

It has been more than 200 years since Doctor James Parkinson's essay on "The Shaking Palsy", where he describes the disease. An excerpt from his paper reads,

"So slight and imperceptible are the first inroads of this malady, and so extremely slow its progress, that it rarely happens that the patient can form any recollection of the precise period of its commencement. The first symptoms perceived are a slight sense of weakness, with a proneness to trembling, most commonly in one of the hands. After a few more months, the patient is found to be less strict than usual in preserving an upright posture. Walking becomes a task which cannot be performed without considerable attention. The legs are not raised to that height, or with that promptitude which the will directs, so that the utmost care is necessary to prevent frequent falls."

Doctor Parkinson's early description of the disease was remarkably accurate, given that he only observed six patients, three of whom he didn't know well, two he encountered on the street, and one he saw from a distance. While not perfect, his description was largely on point. And even after so many years, this description still holds true.

But what about the cure? Is there one?

Unfortunately, there is no cure for Parkinson's Disease as I write this, although tremendous efforts in research and drug trials are ongoing. The truth is that even after more than 200 years of this disease wreaking havoc on those affected by it, scientists and doctors have yet to find a way to fully eradicate the disease. Once diagnosed, you are expected to manage the disease until you die.

But in spite of this, there is hope for those willing to accept Parkinsonism with courage and resilience to make the most out of life despite its challenges. So, the question is, what do you do when this bad news comes knocking on your door?

The answer is simple: *you fight.*

You fight for your rights as a patient, you fight for the best treatments available, and you live life to its fullest despite the hardships that come with it. And you fight for your loved ones who are already in battle. It has been said that when a loved one is affected by Parkinson's, we, in a sense, share the burden. The truth is, Parkinson's disease doesn't just impact those diagnosed; it affects everyone who cares for and supports them, too.

I was a caregiver for my wife, who courageously battled PD for 23 years. During that time, I have had the honor of serving as the President of the local Chapter of the American Parkinson's Disease Association (APDA) for three years and have been a member of their Board of Directors for over a decade. Additionally, my wife co-led a PD support group in Virginia Beach for over ten years. Through these experiences, I have gained a deep understanding of the challenges and hardships that this disease can bring. My journey to creating this guide was rooted in rigorous research, countless conversations, and an unyielding determination to empower those facing the shadows of Parkinson's Disease.

So, how should you approach this guide? Consider it your compass, your steadfast companion. Flip through its pages with an open heart and a curious mind. As you navigate the wealth of knowledge, remember that I stand alongside you, wishing you the best on your journey. In the intricate world of Parkinsonism, where each step can feel like a battle and every movement a conquest, a patient's journey becomes an epic odyssey. This guide illuminates the path ahead, providing not only directions but also the weapons to face the challenges posed by Parkinsonism. From deciphering the symptoms to navigating the treatments, this book serves as a steadfast companion, offering insight and a beacon of hope for those determined to forge ahead.

This book is for the warriors seeking knowledge and empowerment, the families standing strong in solidarity, and the caregivers embracing unwavering support. It's not easy, but with courage, determination, and resilience in your corner – there is always hope. Even with this disease, you can still make the most out of life. You can still enjoy your family and friends, travel, and explore the world - just like anyone else.

If you're ready to forge a path toward clarity and resilience, let's dive in together, armed with understanding and solutions.

Chapter 1: Understanding Parkinson's Disease

Understanding Parkinson's Disease

"I worked in the moving and storage industry for 40-plus years.
Never once did I imagine I would one day be called a "mover" and a
"shaker." –

Mark Colo, author of Peace with Parkinson's.

Your mind is your superpower. The organ with the highest capacity for learning, analyzing, and responding. It's what makes you unique—controlling not only the movement of your body's limbs but every aspect of your life. We go about our daily lives using it to constantly make decisions, interpret information, and control our emotions. Yet, if you have Parkinson's Disease (PD), your mind can feel like an enemy — one that is slowly taking away your ability to think and operate normally.

This disease is so intensely public yet remains largely enigmatic and veiled in mystery. Its effects are many and present differently in each individual. Many of its effects are not confined to private struggles, as they are openly exhibited in the form of immense pain—a pain that cannot easily be masked from the discerning eye. There may be constant movement, shakiness, balance issues, and Dyskinesia. You may slur your speech or speak softer as the years go by. At times, you may feel like you're at war with your own body. It is relentless and can be embarrassing and depressing at times, and for those who have it and their caregivers, it is so very hard.

Parkinson's Disease is the second most common neurodegenerative disease after Alzheimer's; it affects many areas of the nervous system and different types of neurons. Although still not fully understood, it is known that the symptoms of Parkinson's include impaired movement, tremors, slowness or stiffness of movement, slowed speech, and difficulty in walking.

But to understand this long list of symptoms, we must understand what is happening inside the brain. The best way to conceptualize Parkinson's Disease is as one of those diseases of aging, similar to many other age-related conditions. Essentially, as we grow older, various parts of our bodies, including our brains, don't function as efficiently as they used to. Certain areas of our bodies and brains experience deterioration and stop working correctly. Parkinson's Disease involves a specific type of neurological aging that affects certain regions of the brain. It's like aging, but certain parts of your brain are aging more rapidly than the rest of your body.

Causes

The bottom line of this disease is that Parkinson's causes a lack of dopamine, a chemical that controls temperature, mood, movements, and how your brain communicates with every muscle in your body. You're fighting a battle against your brain. Neurons in specific brain regions are affected, particularly the substantia nigra pars compacta in the midbrain. This region is crucial for controlling movement and is where dopamine-containing neurons are located. Parkinson's disease is believed to be caused by a loss of these particular neurons, leading to problems with motor control and coordination.

A distinctive pathology in most cases of Parkinson's is clumps of misfolded proteins within neurons. These clumps, or **Lewy bodies**, are thought to form as a result of specific genetic mutations. A characteristic component of these is a misfolded protein called **alpha-synuclein**. These molecules can form small repeated units called oligomers or longer fibrils. There is mounting evidence to support that these are toxic to neurons and play a key role in driving Parkinson's.

Parkinson's has also been linked to problems with mitochondria. Mitochondria provide cells with the energy to perform vital functions; they are highly dynamic and can fuse together or break up into smaller versions in response to a cell's energy demands. They can also be transported to areas of a cell that need them the most. However, in Parkinson's, these processes can be impaired, and mitochondria are unable to sustain proper neuronal function. As they become old or damaged, mitochondria are removed and replaced. Again, this recycling is thought to be disrupted in Parkinson's, leading to the accumulation of damaged or worn-out mitochondria.

Another idea is that the cells called glia, surrounding neurons, may play a role in Parkinson's. As dopamine neurons are lost, one particular type of glial cell, called microglia, is thought to take up the resulting cellular debris, triggering an immune response. Once activated, they release inflammatory cytokines, which activate neighboring microglia and another type of glial cell called astrocytes. Chemicals released by activated microglia and astrocytes have been shown to injure neurons.

It remains unclear which mechanisms drive the disease process in Parkinson's. What is clear is that with time, more areas of the nervous system develop pathology. To simplify, let me put it this way: *It is a nerve disease of the brain that will get worse with time, guaranteed.*

Risk Factors

There are some risk factors associated with Parkinson's disease that we should consider. Family history plays a role; if you have a parent or child with Parkinson's, your risk is about doubled. However, it's important to note that this might sound like a significant increase, but in the context of the disease's overall rarity, the change in risk is relatively moderate. For instance, instead of having a 1 in 100 chance, it might become a 2 in 100 chance.

Age is a significant risk factor in Parkinson's disease, with the majority of individuals developing symptoms after the age of 60. However, it's worth noting that around 5% to 10% experience onset before age 50. While early-onset forms of Parkinson's may have a hereditary component, it's important to acknowledge that not all cases are inherited. Furthermore, certain gene mutations have been associated with specific variants of the disease.

The risk of Parkinson's disease can also be influenced by **ethnicity** and geographic origin, as certain groups may have a higher predisposition due to genetic factors. A study conducted on 8,514 individuals with Parkinson's disease revealed that 90% were classified as white, 6% as Hispanic, 2% as Asian, and 2% as Black.

Men are more likely to develop Parkinson's than women; the male-to-female ratio is approximately 1.5:1. Pesticides are well-established environmental risk factors, and exposure to them can somewhat elevate the risk. Other environmental toxins, such as industrial solvents, are also associated with a slightly increased risk, although the effect isn't very pronounced.

3

Some intriguing correlations exist, such as the fact that non-smokers appear to have a higher risk of Parkinson's. This could be linked to behavioral traits rather than a direct cause-and-effect relationship. Parkinson's patients are known to display specific personality traits like reliability and caution, which might discourage risky behaviors like smoking. Thus, the smoking-Parkinson's connection could be influenced by factors beyond just smoking itself.

There is also a minor elevated risk associated with a history of concussions. However, it's important to consider that Parkinson's has a long latency period before symptoms become apparent. So, instances, where a concussion occurred may not necessarily be a direct cause but rather an event that occurred after the underlying Parkinson 's-related changes were already underway. In essence, while a connection with concussions exists, it isn't particularly strong, and most individuals who experience concussions won't develop Parkinson's.

Overall, when we look at individual cases, it can be tricky to point out a single cause for Parkinson's. Except for rare genetic instances, chance seems to have a significant role in most cases. Even if you've been exposed to risk factors like pesticides, it's not always the only factor in developing Parkinson's.

Symptoms

Initially, Parkinson's disease was mainly associated with the motor areas of the brain, particularly those responsible for producing dopamine, a neurotransmitter that is deficient in this condition. This dopamine deficiency leads to difficulties in movement, resulting in slow and limited motions. However, it has become evident that the impact of Parkinson's extends beyond just the motor areas. Non-motor areas are also affected, giving rise to a wide range of symptoms. In fact, there is an extensive laundry list of symptoms—around 30 to 50—that can be linked to Parkinson's disease. These symptoms can be related to areas that are closely associated with or located within the same regions of the brain. Let's go through some of these symptoms to gain a better understanding:

Motor Symptoms:

1. **Tremors**, known as rhythmic shaking, typically initiate in a limb, such as your hand or fingers. A common indicator is the thumb and forefinger rubbing together, resembling a pill-rolling motion. Even during rest, the hand may experience

trembling. However, engaging in tasks may alleviate the shaking.

2. Slowed movement, known as **bradykinesia**. As Parkinson's disease progresses, it may gradually slow down your movement, posing challenges in performing daily tasks. Walking might involve shorter steps, and getting up from a chair can become challenging. You may also experience difficulty in lifting your feet and end up dragging or shuffling while walking.

3. Muscle **stiffness** can affect any part of your body, causing discomfort and restricting your range of motion.

4. Sometimes, with Parkinson's disease, you might notice your **posture** becoming stooped or experience balance problems and even falls.

5. You might notice a difference in **automatic movements**. Things like blinking, smiling, or swinging your arms when you walk might not come as naturally as before.

6. **Speech** can vary. You might speak softly or quickly, slur words, or pause before speaking. Your speech may even lack its usual patterns and sound more monotonous.

Non-Motor Symptoms:

1. Reduced sense of smell: Most patients have a decreased or absent sense of smell.

2. Constipation: Common among Parkinson's patients at some point in their illness.

3. Autonomic changes: These include bladder changes, erectile dysfunction, and blood pressure fluctuations upon standing.

4. Sleep disorders: Sleep disturbances like difficulty staying asleep, acting out dreams, and experiencing sleep cycle disruptions. Among the non-motor symptoms are various sleep disorders, each with its own manifestations. These sleep disturbances include difficulty staying asleep, no trouble falling asleep but experiencing difficulty staying asleep, waking up too early, and being unable to return to sleep.

5. In the later stages of the disease, some individuals may encounter problems with movement during sleep, such as acting out their dreams. This can actually serve as an early indication of Parkinson's disease.

6. Psychiatric and cognitive symptoms: Changes in mood, anxiety, and cognitive problems can occur due to imbalances in mood-regulating chemicals.

Cognitive Decline

Generally, older people tend to have a more challenging experience with Parkinson's.

Unlike certain conditions that follow a more predictable pattern, Parkinson's disease exhibits substantial variability. The course it takes depends on multiple factors, including age, individual responses to medication, and the predominance of motor versus non-motor symptoms. It's a complex journey that is unique for each person affected by the disease.

The correlation between Parkinson's disease and dementia is complex. Not everyone with Parkinson's disease will eventually suffer from cognitive decline, but two kinds of cognitive problems can occur in relation to Parkinson's disease.

The first cognitive problem is a sort of **cognitive fog or lack of alertness** that can happen when a person's medications are not effectively managing their Parkinson's symptoms. This can make them feel sluggish, anxious, and less alert. However, this can often be resolved by adjusting medication regimens and through activities like exercise.

The second cognitive issue is the development of **dementia** in some people with Parkinson's disease. This form of dementia is distinct from Alzheimer's disease. It's characterized by difficulties in paying attention, staying focused, and activating memory. While there is a memory deficit, it's not as profound as what is typically seen in Alzheimer's patients. For instance, if you ask a person with dementia associated with Parkinson's to remember a list of words, they might struggle to recall them immediately. Still, they could potentially remember certain details about the words after some prompting. This type of dementia in Parkinson's disease is thought to be related to neurodegeneration occurring in the cortex, the part of the brain responsible for thinking, memory, and concentration. The cognitive challenges often involve difficulties with multitasking, maintaining focus, and experiencing sleepiness.

It's worth noting that not everyone with Parkinson's disease will develop this form of dementia. Additionally, it tends to be more common in older individuals, and it's relatively unusual to experience dementia related to Parkinson's disease at the age of 60 or younger. But if you have Parkinson's for seven years and are 95, you probably will have dementia.

When you look at all these symptoms, it might seem like a long list covering a wide range of potential issues. But it's important to understand that every symptom mentioned directly relates to Parkinson's disease. Different people may experience different combinations of these symptoms, and the severity can also vary.

Diagnosis

With its plethora of presenting symptoms, it should come as no surprise that diagnosing Parkinson's disease is primarily based on pattern recognition and clinical evaluation. It's a process that typically occurs during a doctor's visit and does not require extensive testing. Here's how the diagnosis is made:

First, the doctor diagnoses **"parkinsonism,"** which refers to the presence of slowed movements. This slowing down and stiffness, particularly the hallmark of gradual slowing of movement, are key indicators. If tremors or other characteristic movement abnormalities are observed alongside the slowing and stiffness, parkinsonism is diagnosed.

The next step is determining the underlying cause of this Parkinsonism. In approximately 80% of cases, the cause is Parkinson's Disease, the most common form. However, certain medications, particularly those used to treat conditions like schizophrenia, can induce parkinsonism as a side effect. Additionally, other neurological diseases related to aging might cause similar symptoms. Although not Parkinson's disease, they are treated similarly.

Experienced neurologists can often accurately identify Parkinson's disease based on clinical observations. Sometimes, a member of your healthcare team might recommend a specific type of scan called a dopamine transporter (DAT) scan, which is a single-photon emission computerized tomography (SPECT) scan. The purpose is to gather more information and potentially support the suspicion that you may have Parkinson's disease. It's worth mentioning that not everyone undergoes a DAT scan. Imaging tests, including an MRI, ultrasound of the brain, and PET scans, may be employed to aid in excluding other disorders. Interestingly, these tests are not especially useful in diagnosing Parkinson's disease.

However, researchers are actually looking into a test for Parkinson's that can detect the disease before any symptoms even show up. They're calling it the **alpha-synuclein seed amplification assay**. In a study in 2023, they tested the spinal fluid of more than 1,000 people to see if they could find any clumps of alpha-synuclein, which is found in Lewy bodies. These clumps are a telltale sign of Parkinson's disease. The test had an 87.7% accuracy in identifying people with Parkinson's. It also did a great job detecting those at risk of developing the disease.

Despite the new advancements, a diagnosis might still be unclear, and the doctor will monitor the patient over time. If the condition starts to deviate from the typical progression of Parkinson's disease or if the response to medications is suboptimal, it might indicate another related condition.

Regarding misdiagnosis, it's understandable that stiffness might be mistaken for something like arthritis, especially since you're in your early 50s. However, the distinction lies in the nature of stiffness. In Parkinson's, it's more about an overall movement slowness and difficulty initiating motion rather than localized joint stiffness that you might experience with arthritis.

Ultimately, diagnosing Parkinson's involves a combination of medical tests and clinical observations. Your doctor can order imaging scans to evaluate your brain structure, check your balance and reflexes, as well as observe how you move and respond to medications. In any case, it's important to remain optimistic and stay in contact with your doctor or neurologist about any changes in symptoms or discomfort that you experience. With enough information, you and your doctor can make an informed decision about the best course of treatment.

Progression of Parkinson's Disease

Your battle for control of your body with your brain does not end with a diagnosis. Parkinson's Disease is progressive, meaning it will continue to worsen over time. The progression varies widely among individuals, making it different from many other neurological conditions. There's no single pattern that everyone follows, and Parkinson's is characterized by considerable diversity in its course and evolution.

Many medical professionals who diagnose Parkinson's disease use the Hoehn and Yahr scale to classify symptoms and their severity. So basically, this scale rates the condition and splits it into five stages depending on how the disease progresses. It's a way for doctors to see how far PD has advanced in patients and what treatments might best manage the symptoms.

According to this scale, Stage 1 is the mildest, while Stage 5 is the most severe. Over time, symptoms worsen, and the rate of progression differs between individuals. Some patients spend years in each stage, while others advance to a more severe stage quicker.

The initial phases of Parkinson's disease, often occurring a decade or more before noticeable symptoms, involve subtle changes. Loss of the sense of smell, constipation, and conditions like REM sleep behavior disorder (acting out dreams at night) might emerge during this time. These non-motor symptoms are thought to be caused by the spread of the synuclein protein within the nervous system, even before significant motor symptoms appear.

1. Changes in a Person's Habits

In the early stages of Parkinson's disease (PD), symptoms may appear *mild*, yet they can gradually impact daily tasks and overall quality of life. Although these symptoms may not be overly burdensome, they are certainly present. People around you may observe alterations in movement, note poor posture, and discern changes in facial expressions during this initial phase. Hallmark side effects and symptoms of this stage of Parkinson's disease include **tremors** and other movement issues that tend to be exclusive to one side of the body.

2. Muscle Stiffness and Posture Problems

Stage 2 of Parkinson's disease is often referred to as a *'moderate'* form, where symptoms become more noticeable compared to the previous stage. Notable examples include tremors, stiffness, and trembling. Additionally, facial expression changes may occur, though they might not always be evident to others. It is important to recognize the impact of these symptoms and the need for support and understanding in managing this condition.

In stage 2, you won't typically experience balance problems, but other movement symptoms like muscle stiffness can make tasks a bit more challenging. Plus, you may find that your posture is affected, leading to back and neck pain. At this point, the disease may affect both sides of your body (though usually more on one side), and you might also have some difficulties with speech.

Moving from stage 1 to stage 2 can take months to years, and currently, there's no reliable way to predict how it'll progress. People in stage 2 of Parkinson's disease can usually live independently, but they may find everyday tasks a bit more challenging.

3. Poor Reflexes and Balance Issues

The third stage of Parkinson's is *the mid-point* of disease progression. While some symptoms stay the same or similar to stage 2, stage 3 can bring poorer reflexes and occasional loss of balance. That's why people in this stage may have more noticeable movement issues or seem to slow down. Sadly, falls become more frequent due to balance and reflex problems. Daily tasks become much more challenging at this stage, but people can still live independently. Taking a combination of medication and therapy can help manage the symptoms mentioned earlier.

4. Poor Motor Skills

What sets apart people with stage 3 Parkinson's and stage 4 is their *independence.* At stage 4, motor skills and deep brain stimulation are greatly affected, which in turn affects a person's ability to maintain their independence. Some patients at stage 4 can confidently stand and walk without assistance or equipment, while others may need a walker or similar aids.

Remember, every Parkinson's case is unique. So, it's common for individuals at stage 4 to require assistance and find it challenging to live alone due to the significant impact on their movement and reaction times. Although there may be cases where individuals choose to live alone at this stage, the reality is that daily tasks become extremely difficult and sometimes even dangerous.

5. Severe Stiffness

Stage 5 of Parkinson's disease is the final and most debilitating stage. It's where the disease has advanced the most. At this point, severe stiffness sets in, making it really tough, if not impossible, for a person to stand or walk. Imagine the legs freezing when they try to stand! It's not just difficult but dangerous, too. Daily tasks become impossible without assistance, forcing stage 5 sufferers to rely on wheelchairs. Falling becomes a major concern, so supervision is often necessary.

About 50% of Parkinson's patients in stages 4 and 5 experience confusion, hallucinations, and delusions, with changes in behavior and speech. Depression is also very common at this point due to the amount of physical disabilities and limitations that come with it.

Alternative Scale for Parkinson's Disease

One critique of the Hoehn and Yahr scale is that it only looks at movement-related problems. But we know that PD also brings other symptoms, like different types of cognitive changes and impairment. One example is REM sleep behavior disorder, which can occur as well. That's why some doctors prefer using an alternative called the **MDS-Unified Parkinson's Disease Rating Scale**. This scale has fifty in-depth questions that help analyze both motor and non-motor symptoms. By doing this, doctors can better understand a patient's difficulties, including cognitive function impairments that make daily tasks harder. With this approach, doctors can provide more effective treatments by considering all aspects of a person's condition rather than just focusing on their motor skills.

Diagnosis and Medication Response

After diagnosis, the response to medication becomes a pivotal factor in shaping the disease's progression. Most individuals experience a positive response to medications, often referred to as a "honeymoon" phase. In this period, symptoms are well-controlled, and life carries on with minimal disruptions.

Some individuals, particularly younger ones, might respond exceptionally well to medication. However, over time, managing stable medication doses can become challenging. Symptoms might alternate between being well-controlled and resurging, sometimes with the added complication of dyskinesia, characterized by involuntary movements.

The overall trajectory of Parkinson's is influenced by age. Younger individuals might experience stable symptoms for decades, whereas those in advanced age might face more challenges. Older individuals or those with specific characteristics might experience non-motor symptoms taking the forefront. Sleep disturbances, memory issues, balance problems, and gastrointestinal difficulties might become more prominent.

Treatment Options

Just like the insidious nature of the disease, treatment is a highly individualized process. And to make things clear, it is not "curable." However, medications and lifestyle changes can manage the symptoms of Parkinson's disease to a large extent.

Medical Treatment

In terms of pharmacologic treatments, there are two primary categories of issues to address in Parkinson's disease. One category pertains to motor problems, while the other involves a comprehensive list of non-motor problems. For motor problems, there are several types of medications - dopaminergic agonists, MAO-B inhibitors, anticholinergics, and catechol-O-methyltransferase (COMT) inhibitors. Dopaminergic agents directly stimulate the dopamine neurons and are an essential part of treatment for

Parkinson's disease. They provide symptomatic relief by stimulating the dopamine receptors and can reduce tremors, slow movement, improve posture and coordination, and diminish freezing episodes. MAO-B inhibitors prevent the breakdown of dopamine in the brain, resulting in increased dopamine levels in the brain. Anticholinergics block acetylcholine production, which helps decrease muscle contractions and symptoms such as tremors or rigidity. COMT inhibitors block the breakdown of dopamine in the brain and can improve motor symptoms.

Non-motor treatments encompass a diverse array of options, each tailored to specific challenges. For constipation, there are various approaches available, offering effective solutions. Hyperactive bladder concerns can be addressed with medications that reduce the urge to urinate. Sleep disturbances can be managed with medications and lifestyle changes.

Antidepressants can serve as valuable tools in managing several aspects of Parkinson's disease. They can contribute to improved sleep patterns and help alleviate anxiety. For instance, the persistent worrying about upcoming events, even when there's no apparent cause for stress, is a common feature of Parkinson's disease. Antidepressants can offer relief in such scenarios.

Surgical Avenues

For PD patients experiencing uncontrollable tremors, deep brain stimulation may offer improvement in their quality of life. DBS involves implanting electrodes into certain areas of the brain to help regulate activity in those areas, which can diminish or eliminate symptoms like tremors or stiffness.

DBS is usually offered to people with advanced Parkinson's disease who experience unstable responses to levodopa. It can help stabilize the fluctuations in medicine, reduce or stop involuntary movements (known as dyskinesia), decrease tremors, and improve overall movements. It is effective in controlling the changing responses to levodopa or managing dyskinesia when medication adjustments don't work. However, it's not useful for issues that don't improve with levodopa therapy, except for tremors. Even if levodopa doesn't significantly reduce tremors, DBS can still help control it. Although DBS can provide long-lasting relief for Parkinson's symptoms, unfortunately, it doesn't halt the progression of the disease.

MRI-guided focused ultrasound (MRgFUS) is another treatment that has actually helped some people with Parkinson's disease manage tremors. Basically, it uses ultrasound that is guided by an MRI to target the specific area in the brain where the tremors start. The ultrasound waves then heat up and burn the areas that are causing the tremors. This treatment is still being studied, but the results so far have been promising.

Non-pharmaceutical Treatments

Among the various non-pharmaceutical treatments, one stands out as particularly effective: exercise. Engaging in vigorous exercise, rather than just light walks, has shown to be incredibly beneficial. Furthermore, exercise has been linked to improved sleep quality. In fact, some trials demonstrate its efficacy in enhancing sleep. Additionally, though not definitively proven, there are indications that exercise might slow down the underlying neurodegenerative process. The specific type of exercise may vary based on personal preferences and abilities, but the key is to engage in activities that elevate the heart rate and challenge the body.

Activities like tai chi and dancing can help improve balance, while options like running or swimming are equally valid. The bottom line is to select exercises that push your body, make you feel tired afterward, and raise your heart rate.

Then, there are specific exercises and physical therapies that are specifically designed to address Parkinson's symptoms, like LSVT BIG and PD Warrior. These therapies focus on improving the balance, coordination, and motor performance of those living with Parkinson's. In particular, studies have shown that PD Warrior has resulted in positive outcomes for people dealing with issues related to freezing episodes as well as improved gait and posture. My wife found "BIG" to be an excellent exercise therapy to help her regain some movement control.

When I was President of the local APDA, I saw far too many newly diagnosed individuals. Two pieces of advice I gave to all of them was to get connected to a Parkinson's support group and exercise daily. Don't just sit down and give up...fight! My personal experience is that PD patients, including my wife, who exercised and fought its progression at every stage, had a slower progression. Those who just sat down and gave up usually progressed quickly.

As my wife Zelia used to say, "I may have Parkinson's, but it doesn't have me."

When dealing with a multitude of symptoms, prioritizing and managing treatments can indeed become intricate. The challenge lies in finding the right balance between various medications and addressing side effects, making the expertise of a specialized center crucial, particularly as Parkinson's disease advances.

I hope by now you understand what Parkinson's disease is, how the lack of dopamine can cause different symptoms, how healthcare professionals diagnose it, and the treatments that are available. In the next chapter, we will review the importance of nutrition when living with Parkinson's and how to evaluate diet plans. We will also discuss supplements, vitamins, and how to ensure that you are getting the necessary nutrition for optimal care.

Chapter 2: Nutrition and Diet Guide for Parkinson's Patients and Caregivers

"One thing that I have control over, that makes a difference, is described in the words of Viktor Frankl, who said, "Everything can be taken from a man but one thing: the last of the human freedoms – to choose an attitude in any given set of circumstances." –

Bob Kuhn, diagnosed in 2006

There are only a few things in life that are under your control. Especially if you or someone you love has been diagnosed with Parkinson's, there is only so much you can do to manage symptoms and slow the progression of the disease. What you eat, however, is one thing that is under your control. Before you dive into any new treatment regime, you should know what you're trying to accomplish. If you are trying to treat your symptoms, the treatment may be different than if you are trying to slow Parkinson's disease progression.

One thing already established through years of research is that plant foods like berries may offer protection, and plant-based diets, in general, might help prevent Parkinson's. On the contrary, animal fat and dairy could increase the disease risk. The traditional epidemiologic studies suggest that throughout one's life, in midlife, your 20s, your 30s, your 40s, the more red meat, processed meat, bologna, ham, deli meats, dairy, refined grains, sweets, and desserts, well water, and pesticides you're exposed to, the more likely you are to be diagnosed with Parkinson's disease.

Similarly, in midlife, the more fruits and vegetables, legumes, non-fried fish, coffee, and tea a person drinks, the less likely they are to be diagnosed with Parkinson's disease. And so, naturally, people often wonder, "I read there are five studies that say the more dairy you eat, the more likely you are to be diagnosed with Parkinson's. Should I stop eating dairy?" Or something along the lines of, "I read that green tea protects against Parkinson's disease. I've just been diagnosed. Should I start drinking green tea?"

These are reasonable questions, but before trying to answer these questions, we need to understand why diet matters.

Importance of Proper Nutrition

Gastrointestinal (GI) symptoms can be really bothersome for those with Parkinson's disease. Constipation is the most common symptom, affecting about 80-90% of PD patients. But that's not all. PD's impact on the GI tract doesn't stop there. It can also cause excess saliva (sialorrhea) and swallowing difficulties (dysphagia). And if that's not enough, delayed gastric emptying can lead to those unpleasant feelings of nausea and bloating. So, dealing with the non-motor symptoms of PD can be quite a challenge.

Gut-Brain Connection

Gut dysfunction in Parkinson's Disease (PD) happens for two reasons. Firstly, there's an abnormal accumulation of a protein called alpha-synuclein. It forms clusters called Lewy bodies in neurons responsible for gut function in the lower brainstem, specifically in the dorsal motor nucleus of the vagus.

Additionally, alpha-synuclein also accumulates in structures similar to Lewy bodies in the nerves lining the gut, known as the enteric nervous system (ENS). These Lewy bodies are most common in nerves found in the salivary gland and esophagus. As we move away from the brain, their presence decreases in the gastrointestinal (GI) tract, including the stomach, small intestine, large intestine, and rectum. Notably, the presence of Lewy bodies in the gut can manifest many years before the motor symptoms of PD onset. This helps us understand why constipation is often one of the initial non-motor symptoms experienced in this disease.

Another theory suggests Lewy body pathology starts in the gut and then goes up to the brain through the vagus nerve. They found supporting evidence when they observed that patients who had their vagus nerve cut during surgery for peptic ulcer disease had lower PD rates than the general population. This led to what's now known as the Braak hypothesis, which suggests that over time, Lewy bodies progress within the brain. According to this theory, once the Lewy bodies appear in the lower brainstem, they slowly move up to the midbrain, causing symptoms like rest tremor, slowness, and stiffness commonly seen in PD patients.

Medication Side Effects and the Gut

The relationship between the ingestion of PD medication and the gut can significantly influence motor fluctuations, where a patient's response to Levodopa can vary throughout the day. Gastric emptying delays due to motor symptoms can slow down the absorption of the medication. When medication is taken orally, it may stay in the stomach longer before reaching the small intestine, where absorption happens. This delay in gastric emptying can be a reason why medication doesn't work as effectively.

Protein Effect

Usually, when your doctor prescribes levodopa, they say, "Make sure you take this medicine at least 30 minutes before or a couple of hours after a meal that contains protein." There is a reason for that.

Levodopa actually crosses the wall of the small intestine using a molecule that usually transports amino acids. When there's dietary protein in the small intestine, fewer of these transporters are available for Levodopa to get transported. So, after a protein-packed meal, a patient might feel like the medication isn't working as well. Just remember, dietary protein sources include beef, chicken, pork, fish, eggs, nuts, and dairy.

There are a couple of strategies you can try if you find that your meds are no longer working correctly. One is to avoid protein during the day and instead have it at night, when the medication's impact is less crucial. Another option is to evenly distribute your protein intake throughout the day so that medication absorption remains consistent all day.

The Gut and Inflammation

The immune system protects the body from foreign substances like infections or toxins. Inflammation occurs when the immune system detects a foreign substance, creating a hostile environment to defend the body. While inflammation is necessary to fight attackers, it can sometimes damage healthy tissue, leading to autoimmune diseases like IBD or rheumatoid arthritis.

For three decades, scientists have known that individuals with PD undergo inflammatory changes in their brains. But, recent findings indicate that inflammation isn't just a result of the disease but actually plays a role in its progression. This implies that while the abnormal build-up of alpha-synuclein protein in Lewy bodies might kickstart the disease, it probably triggers an inflammatory response, causing further harm and advancing the condition. Basically, patients with inflammatory bowel disease like Crohn's disease and ulcerative colitis are at a higher risk of developing PD.

The microbiome is the trillions of bacteria, viruses, and fungi that live in our gut. Recent studies have shown that PD patients' microbiome differs from healthy individuals. This suggests that an imbalance in the microbiome could be involved in the development of PD, leading to inflammation in the body.

Recommended Diet for Parkinson's Patients

We all want to decrease symptoms and slow down the progression of PD. But here's the thing: sometimes we have to make trade-offs. If you're 95 years old, then your focus should probably not be on slowing progress. You would want to decrease symptoms.

Now, if you're 45 years old, that's a whole different story. You would want to focus on both decreasing symptoms and slowing progression. So, what diet changes can you make to help reduce the risk of developing PD or slow it down?

Now, I know most of us are used to taking medicine and feeling the symptoms get better in 30 or 45 minutes. That's what we typically think of as symptom improvement. But here's the thing - diet doesn't work that way. You can't just eat some broccoli and expect your rigidity to magically improve half an hour later. And the same goes for a salad or fish, making your tremors disappear. That being said, the impact of diet is more likely to be seen in terms of **non-motor symptoms** and **disease progression**. So, let's see what diets you can follow to reduce your risk of developing Parkinson's disease or slow it down.

Mediterranean diet

A Mediterranean diet is like the diet traditionally eaten in Mediterranean countries. It's all about loads of plant-based goodness like veggies, fruits, whole grains, legumes, and nuts. You'll also find moderate amounts of lean proteins like chicken and fish and fats that revolve around olive oil. Following a Mediterranean diet has been shown to have some impressive benefits for our health. For example, it's been associated with a lower risk of heart disease and even a reduced risk of developing Alzheimer's disease. However, a recent study found that sticking to a Mediterranean diet may also lower the chances of developing prodromal PD. This is a condition where someone doesn't yet meet the motor criteria of PD but has some non-motor features that indicate a higher risk of developing motor PD in the future. It suggests that embracing a Mediterranean diet could potentially delay the onset of PD and slow disease progression.

The MIND diet

The MIND diet is short for Mediterranean Intervention for Neurodegeneration Delay, which is a version of the Mediterranean diet. It focuses on ten super healthy food groups and keeps you away from five not-so-healthy ones.

The ten healthy food groups are:
1. Green leafy vegetables
2. Other vegetables
3. Fish
4. Poultry
5. Beans
6. Whole grains
7. Nuts
8. Berries
9. Olive oil
10. A glass of wine (on a case-by-case basis)

The five unhealthy food groups to be limited include:
1. Red meat
2. Butter
3. Cheese
4. Fried foods
5. Sweets

While the MIND diet may seem strict, there's flexibility in adding variety and incorporating your interests to make it more enjoyable. It's all about finding a proper balance of carbohydrates, fats, and proteins, but with a special focus on being mindful of the sources of fat and carbs, unlike the traditional Western diet.

This diet was initially developed for Alzheimer's prevention and has shown to be effective even if you don't follow it perfectly. It's not about feeling punished but rather seeing it as an opportunity to take proactive steps to prevent the progression of Parkinson's disease. Many patients find the MIND diet empowering as they work towards making positive dietary changes for their health.

Ketogenic Diet

One interesting option is the ketogenic diet, which is low in carbohydrates. This diet promotes the use of ketones as an alternative fuel source, benefiting the brain. An eight-week study showed significant improvements in non-motor symptoms, such as reduced urinary symptoms, pain, fatigue, daytime sleepiness, and cognitive function. While it's important to note that this was a small study involving only five participants, it suggests a promising avenue for dietary modifications in Parkinson's management.

While it's exciting, it's not commonly used in clinics. Firstly, it's highly restrictive. It's already challenging for individuals with Parkinson's to manage their balance, medication timings, and protein intake. Ketogenic diets are known for their strict limitations and lack of sustainability, making them interfere with the overall quality of life. Eating out or enjoying meals with loved ones becomes difficult when following a ketone-friendly diet.

Secondly, ketogenic diets can potentially cause increased weight loss and reduced appetite. Both of these issues are already significant challenges for people with Parkinson's.

Gluten-free diet

A man presenting signs and symptoms of PD but lacking gastrointestinal problems had an unexplained folate deficiency that eventually led to a diagnosis of celiac disease. Treatment for celiac disease involves adhering to a gluten-free diet. The man's vitamin deficiency and PD symptoms improved by adopting a gluten-free diet. This case study supports the notion that some PD patients may benefit from a gluten-free diet.

Usually, a gluten-free diet is recommended for people with celiac disease or gluten sensitivity. If you don't have an allergy, there isn't much evidence to suggest that following this diet would help ease PD symptoms. However, some people find that sticking to a well-thought-out and balanced gluten-free diet improves their quality of life by reducing stomach troubles and fatigue.

These were the specific diet plans that have been linked to a better quality of life in PD patients. But particular foods have also been shown to help people with PD.

Probiotics & Parkinson's Disease

The recognition that the microbiome might have an impact on PD led to the concept that changing the microbiome could potentially alleviate PD symptoms. Probiotics are food or supplements that contain microorganisms (like bacteria or yeast) designed to promote health. As a result, they encompass a broad range of products, including specific yogurts and supplements available in powder or pill form. You can find more information about using probiotics for overall health on the NIH website. Probiotics may function by promoting a harmonious balance of microorganisms in the gut, which is known as the human gut microbiome, and potentially by influencing the body's immune responses.

Although, probiotics have been associated with infections, especially in people with weakened immune systems (like kids or the elderly). But here's the thing: For most people with normal immune systems, taking probiotics usually doesn't cause any trouble, even though we don't have enough scientific evidence to support its widespread use. For example, a clinical trial found that fermented milk used as a probiotic can help manage constipation in PD. But here's the rest of the story - other probiotics haven't been tested as extensively, so we don't really know the best way to treat constipation in PD using this specific pathway.

What we do know is that probiotics could offer potential benefits for a condition called small intestinal bacterial overgrowth (SIBO), characterized by an explosion of bacteria in the small intestine (100-1,000 times the average level). SIBO can lead to symptoms like abdominal pain, bloating, chronic diarrhea, and weight loss. Current studies suggest that this condition is more prevalent in individuals with PD than in the general population and may exacerbate motor fluctuations in PD. By restoring a more balanced bacterial environment, probiotics may help in treating SIBO.

Ultimately, probiotics can offer potential benefits for constipation in PD, but more research is needed to determine the exact role probiotics play in treating this disorder. Additionally, it's important to understand that different probiotic strains and doses may have different effects on constipation in PD, so it's best to withhold experimenting on your own.

Managing Swallowing and Chewing Difficulties

It is incredibly common for people with Parkinson's disease to develop problems with their swallowing and problems with the muscles in their mouth. These muscles control their oral motor skills.

And why is this a problem? There are a couple of significant reasons to consider. Firstly, inadequate nutrition becomes a concern when someone experiences difficulties with eating. This can result in weight loss, which poses a considerable problem. Secondly, and equally important, is the issue of impaired control over food, liquid, and swallowing. This puts individuals at a high risk of aspiration, which occurs when substances other than air enter the lungs. Essentially, anything besides air can cause this problem.

So, if you have PD or you're caring for someone with PD, there are some signs you need to look out for when it comes to oral motor issues:

1. Increased difficulty chewing
2. Problems with tongue control, such as slow speech
3. Difficulty initiating a swallow
4. Coughing while eating or afterwards
5. Continuously clearing throat
6. Taking longer to eat

These can all be indicators of an underlying problem, and if they're present, then seeking medical advice is recommended. There are a range of treatments available that can help people with PD manage their oral motor skills more effectively. Specifically, the healthcare provider that will be addressing that often is a speech therapist. So, if you go to the doctor and are experiencing some of these symptoms, then asking for an evaluation from a speech therapist can be a smart thing to do.

Other helpful tips for maintaining good eating and drinking habits include sitting up straight, taking small bites and sips, focusing on one sip of drink at a time, minimizing distractions while chewing and swallowing, being mindful of fever and cough symptoms, and seeking immediate help when they arise, and consuming food and drink during your medication's "on" period.

When living with Parkinson's, the natural swallowing process tends to slow down, causing saliva to accumulate in the mouth and potentially overflow from the corners. This can occur when your attention is focused on activities like watching TV or carrying out daily chores. Don't underestimate the impact of saliva-related issues. They can result in discomfort, such as cracks forming in the corners of your mouth, leading to difficulties with talking, eating, or drinking. Moreover, these problems can also affect your dental health and increase the risk of mouth infections.

It is important to address these challenges and seek appropriate management techniques. By finding effective solutions, you can improve your quality of life and alleviate any related difficulties. Remember to consciously swallow your saliva regularly and watch out for foods that can make it sticky, like sugary or milky drinks. Discussing medication options with your doctor or a specialist might be helpful if you're dealing with excessive salivation. Here are a few exercises you can try out:

To improve the seal of your lips, just close them as tightly as you can for a count of four, then relax. Repeat this five times.

Give your lips a light smack as if you were puffing on a pipe.

Stretch your lips into a big smile, hold it for a count of four, and then relax.

Purse your lips as if you're going to whistle or kiss someone, hold for a count of four, and then relax.

Again, if you see anything that makes you think that the person you're caring for with Parkinson's disease is having a swallowing problem, it is super important to let the healthcare team know because it can have a severe impact not just on the person's nutrition but on their quality of life. So, it's imperative to address that, and speech therapy is one way to do that.

It's possible to treat dysphagia by adjusting medication and, if necessary, consulting a speech therapist who will suggest a treatment plan to improve swallowing. Try to change your posture when drinking liquids and moisturize drier foods. Be aware of possible signs of dysphagia and always communicate them to the doctor. Never underestimate choking episodes.

In my wife's case, we adjusted for this many times over the 23 years and, toward the end, used thickeners in her drinks and pureed meals to reduce the choking risk.

Dealing With Weight Loss or Gain

Weight changes are relatively common among individuals with Parkinson's disease: some may lose weight, while others might gain. These shifts can impact your overall health. When you're underweight, there's a possibility of reduced muscle mass and strength, increasing your vulnerability to osteoporosis and infection. On the other hand, being overweight raises the risk of heart disease and high blood pressure and adds stress to your joints.

Weight Loss

There are several reasons why people with PD may experience weight loss. Some can lose weight even if they eat the same meals as before, while others might have PD symptoms that affect their appetite or ability to eat.

Gradual loss of smell and taste can diminish the enjoyment of eating. Additionally, feelings of depression or apathy may result in a decreased appetite. Motor symptoms such as tremors, slowness, stiffness, or dyskinesia can make meal preparation and consumption physically challenging. Adjusting PD treatment can be beneficial in these cases. Furthermore, certain PD medications may cause nausea, leading to a reduced appetite, while gastrointestinal issues like constipation, nausea, or bloating can also contribute to decreased appetite.

Swallowing difficulties also interfere with eating. Additionally, some individuals taking levodopa could be advised to limit protein intake with their medications, making it more challenging to receive adequate nutrition throughout the day.

Lastly, severe involuntary movements associated with PD, like dyskinesia or tremors, may increase physical exertion and calorie burn. For example, at one point, my wife experienced a sudden drop in weight over several months. Her nutrition intake was the same, but we were making some medication changes. These changes resulted in increased dyskinesia (body movements) during the medication on and off periods. The neurologist explained that although she was homebound, the dyskinesia had the effect of her running a marathon. The calorie burn was high and resulted in the rapid weight loss. As the medication schedule settled into a correct dosage and interval, the dyskinesia stopped, and her weight returned to normal.

To manage these issues, it is important to be mindful of the foods being eaten and their nutritional content. Research suggests that a diet higher in protein and fiber can help improve motor function associated with PD and improve gastrointestinal symptoms.

There are a few tips to consider to maintain a healthy and balanced diet. Eating small, frequent meals every two to three hours or having nutritious snacks between meals can help keep your energy levels up throughout the day. It's also important to enjoy the foods you eat and have easy-to-prepare options available. Seasoning your food with herbs, spices, and sauces can help stimulate your appetite. Including high-calorie foods like cream and butter (if recommended by your primary care provider) can provide additional nutrients.

If needed, nutritional supplements like Ensure® can be considered. To avoid feeling overly full, it's best to limit consumption of coffee, tea, and clear soups. Additionally, opting for foods that are easy to chew, such as smoothies, ground meats, or other soft proteins, can help prevent fatigue. Don't hesitate to ask for assistance with cutting proteins into smaller pieces if needed.

Weight Gain

On the opposite end of the spectrum, PD patients are also prone to gaining weight. It sounds counterintuitive, but it happens because the body is getting less exercise and has to rely on fat reserves for energy. Over time, this can lead to weight gain.

Not only that, the medications to manage motor symptoms can also cause people to gain weight. Dopamine agonists are medications that are sometimes prescribed alone or with levodopa to help manage the motor symptoms of PD. However, it's important to be aware that they have been associated with compulsive behaviors, like binge eating, which can result in weight gain. If you're experiencing these issues, it's crucial to work closely with your doctor to adjust your medications and address compulsive eating. Simply relying on good intentions alone is unlikely to lead to improvement.

Some medications, particularly those for addressing PD-related psychiatric issues, can cause weight gain. Deep brain stimulation (DBS) can effectively relieve movement symptoms in many individuals; however, it frequently results in weight gain, too.

To combat weight gain, it is recommended to consult a nutritionist or registered dietitian who can assist in developing a healthy, gradual weight loss program. Additionally, eating three nutritious meals a day is essential while being mindful of portion sizes. Avoid excessively strict or low-calorie diets as they may lead to decreased energy levels. Incorporating regular physical activity is crucial, and enrolling in an individual or group exercise program near your home can be beneficial.

Addressing Nutritional Deficiencies

When we talk about the general population, it's clear that elderly individuals are at a higher risk of malnutrition. And you know who else is particularly vulnerable? People who live alone. But here's the thing: those with Parkinson's disease face an even greater risk. We're not entirely sure why. It could be due to apathy, swallowing issues, depression, loss of appetite, or even anorexia. It might also have something to do with malabsorption - where you eat all the right foods, but they're not adequately absorbed. Sadly, malnutrition is pretty common in Parkinson's disease. Depending on the study, anywhere from 25% to 75% of people with Parkinson's are deemed malnourished.

And malnourished people with Parkinson's are more likely to be constipated, depressed, have anxiety, apathy, cognitive impairment, and dystonia muscle pain. Special consideration should be taken to ensure the patient is not deficient in calcium, vitamins D and B12, or iron. Supplements may be necessary if dietary changes are insufficient to meet individual needs.

Antioxidant Foods & Supplements

Essentially, whenever our body goes through some wear and tear, it produces reactive oxygen species and free radicals. Many foods and supplements have antioxidant properties - meaning they can protect against free radicals or reactive oxygen species that can damage cells. A diet packed with fruits, veggies, berries, whole grains, nuts, and seeds tends to be chock-full of antioxidants and is generally believed to provide various health benefits.

Some suggest that an antioxidant-rich diet is good for maintaining optimal brain health in PD, too. However, showing that a specific antioxidant in food or supplements is crucial in preventing or slowing down PD has proven to be quite challenging. Even though it is often talked about, there hasn't been a clinical trial showing that a particular antioxidant protects neurons in PD and is therefore recommended for all individuals with PD.

There are some substances that are currently being studied in clinical trials or have already been studied. However, more data is needed to make recommendations. One of these substances is N-acetyl cysteine (NAC), which works by increasing glutathione levels in the body. Both NAC and glutathione have been studied in relation to PD. Interestingly, glutathione is poorly absorbed through the digestive tract, so two clinical trials have tested intravenous administration of glutathione for PD. These trials showed positive results but were small in scale, and only one included a placebo arm.

We need to do more research with larger groups of patients to find out if this treatment really works. They tried giving patients glutathione through the nose, but it didn't seem to help them more than the placebo. On the other hand, NAC is a supplement taken orally, which might be more promising than glutathione.

Here are some other supplements that are often recommended for Parkinson's disease:

Coenzyme Q10 (Co-Q10)

Research has discovered that individuals with PD may have a deficiency of coenzyme Q10. Although we don't fully understand it yet, we know that coenzyme Q10 plays a crucial role in cellular energy production, neuroprotection, brain function and is a powerful antioxidant.

While some earlier studies raised doubts about the benefits of Coq10 in slowing down the progression of PD, a recent clinical trial revealed that the supplement is safe and well-tolerated by people in the early stages of PD. These findings suggest that it might actually help slow down the advancement of the disease. Another trial is currently underway, which holds promise for early management of PD.

Omega-3 fatty acids

Omega-3 fatty acids are super important for cell growth and muscle activity because they form this protective membrane around neurons. They also help fight inflammation and act as an antioxidant. But our bodies don't make omega-3, so we have to get it from foods (like fatty fish, think salmon) or supplements. Other sources of omega-3 include flax seeds, walnuts, and chia seeds.

A study in 2020 found that omega-3 might actually help improve motor skills in people with PD by protecting brain health and reducing inflammation. That said, while omega-3 fatty acids could be helpful for someone with PD, we don't have solid evidence that they can extend life.

Creatine

Creatine is known for its ability to activate ATP (adenosine triphosphate), providing the energy necessary for muscle and brain tissue. It's commonly used in the sports world to enhance performance. When it comes to PD, some studies suggest that taking creatine early in the disease may help slow down progression. However, other studies have yet to show any noticeable benefit. In fact, a study analyzed five randomized control trials with 1339 participants and found no evidence of creatine being beneficial for people with PD.

Vitamin B12

Vitamin B12 plays a vital role in protecting and supporting the function of nerve cells, as well as in the production of red blood cells. However, individuals with PD and older adults often have low levels of vitamin B12. Several studies suggest that low levels of this vitamin may increase the risk of developing PD. Moreover, the use of levodopa can hinder the body's ability to absorb and utilize folic acid, folate, and vitamin B12, leading to elevated levels of homocysteine. The duration and dosage of levodopa treatment directly impact the levels of homocysteine, and high levels of this compound have been linked to adverse outcomes in individuals with Parkinson's.

Although there isn't concrete evidence linking B12 to longevity, it can certainly enhance your quality of life. So, it's worth considering B12 supplementation. But before jumping on any specific method, like oral tablets or injections, it's best to consult your healthcare provider. They might want to run a lab test to check your B12 levels first.

Vitamin C

Vitamin C, an essential antioxidant, plays a crucial role in protecting neurons from cell damage caused by free radicals. While citrus foods are a good source of this vital nutrient, many adults do not consume enough whole foods to meet their requirements. Supplementation becomes necessary, especially for individuals with Parkinson's disease, who often have lower stomach acid levels. Roughly 58% of Parkinson's patients experience hypochlorhydria, a condition characterized by insufficient stomach acid production. This can hinder the absorption of nutrients from food and impede the effectiveness of medications. To optimize levodopa absorption, it is often recommended to take it with either 30 ml of lemon juice or a 500 milligram powdered vitamin C packet. This will enhance the availability of levodopa in each dosage.

Furthermore, clinical trials have shown that supplements such as Vitamin E do not provide benefits for Parkinson's disease (PD). However, while showing promise in pre-clinical models, substances like curcumin and tauroursodeoxycholic (TUDCA) require further study in humans before they can be recommended for use in PD.

Alternative Supplements and Treatment

Continuous advancements are being made in the area of alternative treatment and supplements for PD. There are some other ongoing therapies or supplements that are being considered to slow disease progression or improve symptom management. Some of these are:

Coffee & Tea

Many studies have actually shown a link between caffeine consumption and a lower risk of PD. And get this: these studies have found this connection when looking at various dietary sources like coffee, black tea, green tea, and overall caffeine intake. Coffee has the potential to protect against Parkinson's development and progression. Studies even suggest that Parkinson's patients who drink coffee or caffeinated tea might reduce their risk of premature death by half. But remember, correlation doesn't always mean causation.

Researchers are studying whether other substances, like caffeine and Eicosanoyl-5-hydroxytryptamine (EHT), may play a role in reducing the risk of PD. Dr. M. Maral Mouradian, interim director of one of APDA's Centers for Advanced Research at Rutgers-Robert Wood Johnson Medical School, conducted research that showed how caffeine and EHT may work together to prevent biochemical changes associated with the development of PD. While further research is needed to test these compounds in humans and determine the required amount for the protective benefit, the findings suggest that coffee might have beneficial effects.

Green and black tea have all these substances with antioxidant properties that seem to protect neurons in cell culture and animal models. But we're still determining if the same effects happen in people when they drink tea. One study found that only black tea, not green tea, reduced the risk of Parkinson's disease compared to just caffeine. So, maybe black tea has something extra besides caffeine that affects PD risk. We need more research to determine how tea lowers PD risk and what doses will work.

It's still unclear whether caffeine, coffee, or tea can actually be helpful for someone who already has PD. Apart from the fact that they've been associated with a lower risk of developing PD, could caffeine actually help with PD symptoms?

Different studies come to different conclusions. In one, they gave people with PD caffeine as a symptomatic medication, but it didn't benefit motor symptoms. However, another study found that people with PD who consumed more caffeine had better motor and non-motor scores during the first four years after diagnosis.

To dig deeper into the effects of caffeine, researchers conducted a study called "Caffeine for the treatment of Parkinson's disease." They started the caffeine group with a dosage equal to a cup of coffee twice daily, then gradually upped it to two cups daily. That's like four cups of black tea or six cups of green tea. And within just three weeks, the caffeine group showed significant improvement in Parkinson's symptoms compared to the placebo group.

So, it seems like there's still more research to be done before we can say for sure whether your morning coffee or tea actually makes a difference once you've been diagnosed with PD.

Velvet beans

We know most of the symptoms of PD are a manifestation of low dopamine levels in the brain. Now, while foods rich in dopamine don't really help because of the blood-brain barrier, there's this thing called levodopa that can enter the brain and get converted into dopamine. We use decarboxylase inhibitors to ensure dopamine is produced in the brain and not anywhere else.

Even though levodopa is the standard treatment for Parkinson's, it's not cheap. In some low-income areas, like rural Africa, it costs about a dollar daily. That's a lot, so only a few patients can afford it. An Indian physician found that velvet beans have a lot of L-DOPA so they could be a treatment option. Velvet beans have been used as an alternative or supplement to Levodopa in places where the drug isn't available or affordable. Clinical studies suggest that velvet beans can provide a reliable and long-lasting antiparkinsonian effect, working even faster and better than the drug itself!

In a study with advanced Parkinson's patients, they switched between roasted velvet bean powder and the standard drug. And guess what? They observed changes in their quality of life, daily activities, movement symptoms, and mobility. It turns out that velvet beans showed similar effectiveness as the drug, which hints at their potential as an alternative therapy for Parkinson's disease.

Of course, Levodopa in pill form should still be the primary treatment for Parkinson's. But velvet bean powder might be better tolerated by certain patients, especially those who aren't fans of pills. However, let's remember that using velvet bean supplements comes with challenges commonly associated with all supplements, including the lack of regulation and quality control issues. Out of the six brands they tested, four showed significant discrepancies between labeled and actual L-DOPA content.

Even though the inexpensive herbal remedy from velvet beans is effective, there are practical reasons why it probably won't be licensed. First, the remedy's taste could be better, and we only have a little data on its long-term effects beyond a few months. While velvet beans might potentially treat Parkinson's disease in low-income countries, experts advise against using them instead of drugs in wealthier nations.

Fava Beans

Fava beans also offer a natural source of L-DOPA. Although they contain about ten times less L-DOPA than velvet beans, their quantity in food form can compensate for the difference. Fava beans have enough L-DOPA to be pharmacologically active in Parkinson's disease, and some reports suggest patients might respond better to them than pill-form L-DOPA.

It's remarkable how fava beans can actually have similar levels of L-dopa as drug formulations, even though they don't contain the carbidopa booster. It turns out that fava beans might naturally provide both L-dopa and carbidopa. So, if you eat fava beans, it can increase the levels of L-dopa and carbidopa in your blood, which can lead to some pretty significant improvements in muscle movement for Parkinson's patients.

Despite the potential benefits, there are certain drawbacks associated with fava bean consumption. Notably, fava-induced flatulence, interactions with MAO inhibitor drugs used for depression, and the risk of favism—a genetic mutation that hinders the detoxification of compounds in fava beans and can cause red blood cells to rupture. Genetic testing for this mutation is recommended before considering daily fava bean consumption.

For those interested in trying fava beans, fresh green ones contain more L-dopa than dried beans. Roasting and boiling can diminish L-dopa content, though cooked favas still offer around 250 mg per half cup. Sprouted favas may provide the most L-dopa, particularly after day 9 when indigestible sugars decrease due to sprouting.

Research has shown promising results with fava bean sprouts. Feeding Parkinson's patients a salad containing half a cup of freshly chopped fava sprouts resulted in significant clinical improvement. Other beans, including soybeans, also contain L-DOPA, albeit in lower amounts. Soybeans additionally possess a compound that might act as an L-dopa-boosting carbidopa compound. A study found that giving people a small portion of roasted soybeans alongside their regular Parkinson's medications led to significant improvement and fewer involuntary movements compared to drugs alone.

Other than these, eating more foods rich in antioxidants and omega-3s, as well as reducing saturated fats, are beneficial for people with Parkinson's. Flaxseed is especially recommended due to its high levels of omega-3 and antioxidants. A study found that eating flaxseed supplementation significantly improved motor scores in Parkinson's patients over six months. Additionally, correcting any nutrient deficiencies may help alleviate some Parkinson's symptoms.

The diet for a person with PD is not one size fits all. Everyone is different and may have various sensitivities to foods and ingredients, so it's essential for each individual to find the ideal diet that works best for them. Finding your particular diet or one that suits the person you are a caregiver for can be challenging. The amount of sleuthing and research needed to find the perfect dietary fit for PD can be overwhelming.

To differentiate and personalize your diet, the best method you can use is keeping a food diary. A food diary helps you see which foods may be affecting motor scores positively or negatively by tracking what you eat and observing the changes in your motor scores. By making careful dietary adjustments and keeping track of your food, you can find a diet that works best for you or the person with PD you are caring for.

No matter what diet you decide is right for you, it's important to ensure your meals are balanced and nutritious. Making lifestyle changes can be challenging, so finding ways to make healthy eating habits easier and more enjoyable is essential. Eating meals together as a family or with friends can help keep everyone motivated when trying new recipes or healthy snacks. It is also beneficial to focus on one small change at a time so that you can more easily track and adjust any changes in motor scores. Finally, remember that everyone's needs are different when it comes to diet and nutrition.

In the next chapter, we will delve deeper into another form of lifestyle change: exercise. We will explore the benefits of exercise and discuss how to incorporate it into your lifestyle in a healthy and sustainable way.

Chapter 3: Exercise and Physical Therapy Guide for Parkinson's Patients and Caregivers

"Today, in comparison to eight years ago, I am now taking about half the amount of medication that I used to. My exercise program has not only halted the progression of my condition, but it has also effectively given me back a few years that I may have otherwise lost."
—Jimmy Choi, diagnosed with Parkinson's at age 27, Guinness World Record holder for highest number of chest-to-ground burpees in one minute.

The act of exercising can not only be a helpful way to manage symptoms but also aid in slowing down and possibly reversing the progression of Parkinson's disease over time. Since PD is an evident motor disorder characterized by rigidity, tremors, and impaired balance, exercise can help improve these symptoms.

Currently, over 2,000 research papers focus on the relationship between Parkinson's disease and exercise, and this number continues to grow steadily. The encouraging news is that there are presently 137 ongoing trials dedicated to further establishing a solid evidence base for the benefits of exercise. It is a widely shared belief that exercise indeed holds significant positive effects.

Benefits of Exercise for Parkinson's Patients

Daniel Corcos, Ph.D., who has been studying the effects of exercise on people with Parkinson's disease since 2001, found that Progressive resistance exercise has been shown to reduce the symptoms of Parkinson's disease significantly. As a result of specific exercise protocols, participants became stronger and faster, and their muscle activation patterns improved, leading to increased satisfaction and well-being.

In the Study in Parkinson's Disease of Exercise Phase 2 (SPARX2), 128 early PD patients not yet on medication were divided into three groups:

1. High-intensity treadmill exercise (80-85% max heart rate)
2. Moderate-intensity treadmill exercise (60-65% max heart rate)
3. Wait-list control group

After six months, the high-intensity group showed minimal change in motor scores, while the control group worsened by three points.

One of the main benefits is that it can improve balance, coordination, flexibility, and strength in muscles affected by PD's motor symptoms. Other advantages include improved gait speed as well as increased psychological well-being through social activities as opposed to sitting idle at home. This shows that exercise can **slow down the progression** of PD, allowing patients to gain greater control of their lives.

However, the most significant changes have been found related to physical exercise's effects on the brain. Researchers at the University of Southern California looked at the brains of mice that had exercised under conditions parallel to a human treadmill. They discovered that exercising doesn't actually change the amount of dopamine in your brain, but it makes the brain cells **use dopamine more efficiently**. So, it improves efficiency by tweaking the parts of your brain that receive dopamine signals - the substantia nigra and basal ganglia.

Scientists at the University of Pittsburgh discovered that exercise has a positive impact on the brain by increasing beneficial neuron growth factors. Specifically, it boosts GDNF (glial-derived neurotrophic factor), which helps protect dopaminergic neurons from damage. This finding suggests that exercise might help reduce inflammation in the brain, which is important because inflammation is thought to play a role in the development of Parkinson's disease. Moreover, individuals with PD who begin exercising earlier in their disease journey, dedicating a minimum of 2.5 hours per week, notice a **slower decline in their quality of life** compared to those who start later.

In summary, higher levels of physical activity are associated with **lower mortality rates**. In practical terms, this translates to approximately about five to nine hours of moderate-intensity activities per week. Coupled with a healthier diet, these habits appear to positively impact mortality, and these findings apply both before and after diagnosing a condition.

Types of Exercises for Parkinson's Patients

Now that we know that physical activity is beneficial for Parkinson's patients, you should know that asking for a referral for physical therapy is the way to go. A physical therapist will be able to figure out what movement challenges you may have and design a program to help you improve.

An exercise program should be made of four key components. The first component is **aerobic fitness**, involving activities like bicycling, rowing, or brisk walking. The second component is **strengthening**, which can be achieved through weight machines or small weights. The third component is **stretching.** Yoga can be particularly beneficial for this. The fourth and crucial component is **agility**, which focuses on balance and fall prevention.

Engaging in at least 30 minutes of exercise daily on at least five days of the week is recommended for optimal results. And while incorporating all four components into each day is ideal, you can tailor your routine by dedicating specific days to different aspects of exercise.

Aerobic Exercise

The aerobic exercise you choose should be enough to get your heart rate up and increase your need for oxygen. Make sure you sustain the activity for more than 10 minutes at a time and do it multiple times throughout the week. Here are some practical tips to guide your aerobic activity:

According to the CDC, older adults (who are generally fit) should aim for 150 minutes of moderate-intensity exercise or 75 minutes of vigorous-intensity exercise every week. What does that mean? Well, during moderate-intensity exercise, you should be able to talk but not sing - you'll be a bit winded. But during vigorous-intensity exercise, you should only be able to say a few words before pausing for a breath.

Notably, high-intensity interval training (HIIT) is an exercise where you go all out for short bursts and then take it easier for a bit. It's gotten pretty popular, and some studies even suggest it has more health benefits compared to keeping a steady pace. Some smaller studies have also shown that this kind of workout could be beneficial for PD, too.

Stretching

Muscle stiffness for patients with PD is one of those things that don't have an easy fix. Stretching can help, but it's not just about making your muscles feel less tight. A good stretching routine should also help improve coordination and balance - which are both common issues with PD patients. It is often the muscles that control joint movement that tend to tighten in individuals with Parkinson's disease. As a result, the Parkinson's Foundation advocates for a stretching routine that emphasizes these areas:

1. Shoulders and elbows
2. Calves
3. Hamstrings and knees
4. Wrists and palms
5. Lower back
6. Neck
7. Chest wall

Flexibility is crucial for everyday movements like walking, bending, and lifting. By incorporating stretching exercises, you'll find it easier to get out of bed, dress yourself, grab items from the floor, and complete other tasks. So, if you want to improve your flexibility, simply share your desired areas with your physical therapist, and they'll guide you through targeted stretches for those muscles.

Strength Training

It is very easy to feel like you cannot hold your own while doing everyday things because it is one of those things that keeps one independent. Holding your brush, putting on a hair tie, and lifting the book you had been reading off the floor are activities that require strength. Both Parkinson's disease and the natural process of aging can result in muscle weakness if you don't keep up with strength training. The good news is there are various ways to strengthen your muscles, such as lifting weights, using resistance bands, or even just using your own body weight. So, no matter what stage of Parkinson's you're in, you can still make those muscles stronger.

To make the most of your progress and focus on specific areas, your trusted physical therapist will choose safe and effective strength training exercises. These exercises will not only improve your posture, endurance, and motor symptoms but also cater to your personal goals and needs.

Make sure to have open communication with your therapist and share your objectives so they can provide personalized guidance. For example, if you find it difficult to stand up from a chair, your therapist can help strengthen your leg muscles. Or, if you're having trouble with handwriting, your therapist can focus on exercises to improve hand dexterity. Your physical therapist will also provide feedback and track your progress over time to ensure that the exercises are working for you. With their help, you can work towards providing relief from motor symptoms and improving overall muscle strength. So don't hesitate – start slowly with low-intensity exercises and find the right therapist to work on your specific goals.

Dual-Task Practice

Even if it sounds easy to do, dual-task practice can be challenging to execute. It's a combination of physical and cognitive activities that involve performing two different tasks simultaneously.

Multitasking or transitioning between tasks can be difficult for individuals with Parkinson's. This can increase the risk of falling and make everyday activities more challenging. If you struggle with multitasking, your physical therapist may suggest practicing two activities simultaneously to address this symptom. Doing this type of exercise with your therapist can help you become more aware of how you move, provide insight into task performance, and enable better coordination between your brain and body.

As an example, you may be asked to perform activities like counting while walking, bouncing a ball, or identifying objects. The objective is to train your brain to multitask effectively. Engaging in dual-task practice can also improve your balance abilities.

There's actually evidence to suggest that adding a cognitive aspect to exercise, like picking up a new motor skill, can be really helpful for people with Parkinson's. That's why activities such as boxing, dancing, tai chi, or yoga have gained popularity among those with PD. These kinds of activities help individuals become more aware of how they're moving, provide insight into task performance, and enable better coordination between the brain and body.

Karate and Golf have also been especially helpful for those with PD as they both involve motor skills and cognitive aspects. Karate helps to improve balance, posture, coordination, and reaction time. And in golf, the physical aspect of swinging a club works together with the mental challenge of strategizing and focusing on each shot.

Physical Therapy Techniques for Parkinson's Patients

After exercise, physical therapy is a great way to help control Parkinson's symptoms. Specific techniques can be used to improve movement capabilities. A therapist also helps individuals with PD develop better posture and more efficient ways of doing everyday tasks such as cooking or dressing oneself.

Amplitude Training

A specific and highly effective form of physical therapy for individuals with Parkinson's disease is known as LSVT BIG training. LSVT, which stands for Lee Silverman Voice Treatment, encompasses innovative techniques to address various symptoms associated with the condition. LSVT LOUD, for instance, concentrates on voice amplification therapy. In the case of LSVT BIG, the focus is on enhancing the "amplitude of movement" in Parkinson's patients.

During LSVT BIG training, patients engage in exaggerated physical movements, such as high steps and arm swings. These intentional actions aim to retrain the muscles and counteract the progression of hypokinesia - a hallmark of Parkinson's characterized by gradually diminishing and shuffling movements. By incorporating LSVT BIG into a comprehensive treatment plan, individuals can potentially slow down the advancement of the disease.

An example of an amplitude training exercise is the Toe-Tap. For this particular exercise, patients must lift their toes as high as possible and then quickly tap them onto the ground. Over time, this can help improve the ability of a patient to walk more regularly with less effort. Other exercises used in LSVT BIG include trunk rotations, arm circles, shoulder shrugs, and leg swings.

Reciprocal Patterns

Reciprocal movements refer to side-to-side and left-to-right patterns, such as the natural swinging of your arms while taking steps during a walk. These patterns may be impacted by Parkinson's disease, affecting mobility and coordination. In order to reinforce and improve these reciprocal patterns, your therapist may suggest incorporating exercises with specific equipment such as a recumbent bicycle - a stationary bike where you sit in a reclined position or an elliptical machine - which engages both your arms and legs.

Furthermore, you can also practice on your own by focusing on walking with the intention of maintaining the swinging motion of your arms. To help keep a consistent rhythm, it may be beneficial to chant or sing while you walk. Additionally, exploring activities like dance classes or tai chi can be advantageous in promoting and enhancing reciprocal movements. By incorporating these strategies into your routine, you can actively work towards improving the coordination and rhythm of reciprocal movements, ultimately supporting your overall mobility and well-being.

Balance Work

Normal balance is a complex interplay of various factors. It involves visual feedback, where your eyes help you perceive your surroundings; your inner ear, which assists in orienting yourself, and the sensory input from your feet, allowing you to perceive the ground beneath you.

In the case of Parkinson's disease, this delicate balance system can be disrupted, leading to an unstable gait and a sense of fear when in public or crowded spaces. Gait training, which involves practicing walking, can be highly beneficial in improving this condition. It is advised to seek the guidance of a physical therapist who can thoroughly assess your balance issues and provide personalized exercises to address them. With their expertise, they can help you understand the underlying causes and teach you practical strategies to compensate for any balance impairments. It is true that no one knows your disease better than yourself, and with the proper guidance and determination, you can make great strides to improve your gait and feel confident in any situation.

Apart from physical therapy, there are a few steps that you can take in order to try and get better at walking:

1. Ensure you have suitable footwear with enough cushioning around the feet.
2. Set realistic goals for yourself and break them into smaller, achievable goals you can work towards.
3. Pay attention to your form when you are walking; keep your head up, back straight, and arms bent at the elbows.
4. Make sure you are taking plenty of breaks and use a cane or walker to help with stability while walking.
5. Practice exercises that focus on balance, coordination, and proper gait mechanics.
6. Consider using an orthotic device such as a brace or shoe insert to help with support and stability.

Being consistent with your walking practice will help you to become more comfortable and confident in your ability to walk. Walking for at least 30 minutes a day can also help improve your overall health and fitness. Additionally, do not forget to be safe while walking, as this can help you avoid falls or injuries. In my experience as a caregiver, as my wife's falls and freezing episodes increased, I held on to her arm everywhere we went. It allowed me the opportunity to catch her if she fell and saved us many potential injuries.

Adaptations for Different Stages of Parkinson's Disease

Just like the flow of time, PD is a disease that does not stand still; it is progressive. As the disease progresses, you may experience different symptoms that require different approaches to your exercise regimen.

Understanding the progression of Parkinson's disease and distinguishing its stages can enable patients and caregivers to anticipate evolving needs, access appropriate support, and make informed decisions about treatment and lifestyle adjustments. By recognizing the specific symptoms and challenges associated with each stage, individuals can proactively manage the impacts of the disease and enhance the overall quality of life.

In the early stage, patients may experience subtle changes, such as slight tremors and alterations in gait, posture, and facial expression. These symptoms often go undiagnosed as they do not significantly interfere with daily life. During stage two, tremors become more pronounced and affect both sides of the body, accompanied by a sense of rigidity. Walking and posture issues become noticeable during this stage.

The exercise of choice during the early stages of Parkinson's should focus on strength, balance, flexibility, and overall coordination. As the disease progresses, aerobic activity should be introduced. However, if physical functioning becomes limited, activities such as tai chi and yoga may be beneficial. It is essential to ensure that exercises are adapted to meet the needs of each individual.

During stage three, mobility becomes increasingly difficult and is accompanied by freezing, which occurs when a person experiences difficulty initiating or continuing movement. The risk of falling increases during this stage, so special attention should be paid to balance exercises.

In the later stages of Parkinson's, physical activity becomes more limited and poses an increased risk of injury. Low-impact exercises such as swimming, chair yoga, tai chi, or walking can help improve quality of life. Exercise should be tailored to the individual needs of each person with Parkinson's to maximize its benefits.

It is also important for individuals with Parkinson's to remain socially active throughout their journey. Connecting with other people diagnosed with the condition can provide invaluable support, as can joining social activities in the local community.

Finally, it is important to remember that everyone's experience of Parkinson's disease is unique, and what works for one person might not work for another. It is, therefore, essential that people with Parkinson's and their caregivers regularly assess the treatments that are most effective for them, making sure to consult a healthcare professional when needed. One thing that should be of note is to know your limitations and needs regarding the condition. People must refrain from over-exerting themselves, as this can have a negative impact on their health.

Here are some important safety tips to keep in mind during your exercise routine:

1. Take your Parkinson's medication 30 minutes to an hour before starting your exercise session. This can help improve mobility and reduce the risk of experiencing symptoms during the workout.
2. If you find it challenging to perform exercises independently or experience difficulty, consider having a caregiver accompany you during your workout. Their support can ensure your safety and provide assistance if needed.

Stop exercising if you encounter these conditions:

1. Frequent freezing of gait: Difficulty with movement and high risk of falls.
2. Low blood pressure after Parkinson's medication: Significant drop in blood pressure after medication.
3. Abnormal heart rate response: Unusual changes in heart rate during exercise.

By incorporating these different types of exercises into your routine, you can enhance your overall physical fitness, improve balance and flexibility, and support your health and well-being. Remember to tailor your exercise plan to your individual needs and abilities, and consult with a healthcare professional if you have any underlying health conditions or concerns.

In the next chapter, we will review all the current medications used to manage PD symptoms, how they act, and how to take them to get the best results.

Chapter 4: Medication Management Guide for Parkinson's Patients and Caregivers

"Find something that is your cause, what you want to stand up for in life, and stand up for it. Mine is slightly narcissistic because it's Parkinson's. I mean, that's ridiculous. I should have other causes that I look up to as well. But before I was diagnosed, I didn't fight for anything. Now, I fight for my own life, my own existence, and what I want to do in my life. And I fight for others." - Diagnosed with Parkinson's at 29, Emma Lawton has written about her experience in her book, Dropping the P Bomb.

We are living in a day and age when there is a dizzying array of drugs available, and the sheer number can be overwhelming. Effectively managing Parkinson's disease can present intricate challenges, including the precise administration of a variety of medications at designated times. At first, treatment may seem relatively straightforward, involving three daily doses of medication. However, as the disease advances, navigating the disease can become increasingly complex.

The goal of this chapter is to provide some direction and guidance on how to best manage medication for Parkinson's patients and their caregivers. We'll discuss developing a medication management plan, the importance of communication between patient and doctor, understanding drug interactions, taking medications safely, and tracking drug effectiveness.

The choice of medication for treating Parkinson's disease is not one-size-fits-all and depends on various factors. These factors include the severity of symptoms, whether the symptoms affect the dominant or non-dominant hand, how symptoms impact work and activities, the effect on daily living tasks, and the financial considerations. It's important to note that this decision-making process is a collaborative effort between you and your neurologist. Together, you will discuss and determine the most appropriate treatment approach based on your circumstances.

Commonly Prescribed Medications

As with any disease, we know there is a baseline dysfunction that manifests in the body. In Parkinson's, we know it is the low level of dopamine in the brain. As a result, medications and therapies are aimed at restoring dopamine balance or replacing it with something similar to help restore movement. However, dopamine can't be given directly because it can't enter the brain. Therefore, doctors prescribe drugs that either mimic dopamine or increase levels of dopamine in the body.

Levodopa and carbidopa

Central to treating Parkinson's disease is levodopa, an invaluable form of dopamine. Commonly prescribed as "Sinemet," this remarkable treatment is highly effective. In fact, for most individuals with Parkinson's disease, levodopa becomes an indispensable component of their treatment regimen, often initiated in the early stages of the disease.

In essence, levodopa helps compensate for the dopamine deficiency and significantly improves motor symptoms associated with Parkinson's disease. It's a crucial therapeutic tool that plays a central role in managing the condition. It primarily targets symptoms such as bradykinesia (slow movement) and rigidity. It can significantly improve daily activities such as morning preparation, changing, bathing, and eating. However, its effectiveness on tremors and freezing of gait can vary among individuals.

Levodopa works by being converted into dopamine by your brain cells, helping to alleviate the symptoms of Parkinson's disease. Sinemet, on the other hand, is a combination of levodopa and carbidopa. Adding carbidopa enhances levodopa's effectiveness, allowing for a lower dosage and reducing the likelihood of common side effects like nausea, vomiting, and irregular heart rhythms. This combination therapy provides a more targeted and efficient approach to managing Parkinson's symptoms.

Sinemet, a commonly prescribed medication for Parkinson's disease, is known for having the fewest short-term side effects compared to other treatment options. However, it is important to note that long-term use of Sinemet may increase the risk of developing involuntary movements, which can be a significant concern.

Individuals who have been taking levodopa for 3-5 years may begin experiencing restlessness, confusion, or dyskinesia shortly after consuming the medication. Orthostatic hypotension, a type of low blood pressure caused by standing up quickly that can cause dizziness and fainting, may also occur. Managing OFF periods is essential to help individuals remain symptom-free for as much of the day as possible. Various strategies are available to address OFF periods, including changing the timing or dosage of levodopa/carbidopa, taking rest breaks, eating small, frequent meals, or adding other medications that may help reduce OFF periods.

In my wife's case, the need for Sinemet adjustments became more common as her journey progressed. This is due to the treatment window narrowing. An adjustment of dosage or frequency was often needed when her reaction to the medication would change.

How To Take Levodopa

When taking immediate-release levodopa, it's a good practice to make it the first thing you consume in the morning. Place the tablet next to your bed with a small glass of water. By the time you're up, brushed, and prepared for the day, the medication will have around 30 minutes to take effect. This way, you can start your day feeling the benefits of the medication. For instances where you may need levodopa during the night, it's recommended to use the immediate-release formulation. If you're having trouble falling back asleep, chewing the tablet and taking it with a carbonated beverage can help speed up its onset of action.

Controlled-release levodopa is often used at bedtime to manage symptoms throughout the night. It can help prevent sleep disruptions caused by repositioning difficulties or other Parkinson 's-related issues. Discuss your experiences with your neurologist and inform them of any changes in your nighttime symptoms to ensure the best treatment plan.

It is best absorbed on an empty stomach, which helps enhance its absorption. Taking levodopa about 30 to 60 minutes before meals and 1 to 2 hours after meals is generally recommended. Some sources suggest 60 minutes before meals and 2 hours after meals. However, taking it 30 minutes before meals and waiting a bit longer after meals (up to 2 hours) is also acceptable. The key is to find a timing that works best for you and is easy to follow.

When taking levodopa, it's important to space it apart from certain substances that could interfere with its absorption. Iron supplements should be spaced apart by at least two to three hours from your levodopa dose. This is to avoid any potential interaction that could reduce the absorption and effectiveness of levodopa.

Additionally, it's crucial to avoid taking levodopa with protein-rich foods or supplements, as protein can compete for absorption at the same site and potentially reduce the effectiveness of levodopa. To prevent this competition, taking levodopa on an empty stomach helps ensure it's absorbed efficiently without interference from protein. Ultimately, the goal is to optimize the absorption of levodopa and ensure you receive the maximum benefit for symptom management. If you have any concerns or specific dietary restrictions, I would suggest you discuss the timing and considerations for taking levodopa with your healthcare provider.

Dopamine Agonists

These medications, like pramipexole (Mirapex), rotigotine (Neupro), and ropinirole (Requip), mimic dopamine's effects in the brain. Amantadine (Gocovri, Osmolex ER, Symmetrel), may offer relief for individuals with mild Parkinson's disease by increasing dopamine availability in brain cells and reducing symptoms. Recent studies even suggest that amantadine can help with the involuntary movements that come with levodopa therapy.

For the treatment of Parkinson's disease, you have the option to take one of these drugs individually or in combination with Sinemet. In some cases, doctors may initially prescribe dopamine agonists and then introduce levodopa if symptoms remain uncontrolled. Dopamine agonists are often preferred as a first-line treatment due to their lower risk of long-term complications compared to levodopa therapy. Dopamine agonists can cause hallucinations, increased confusion, and the development of compulsive behaviors, especially at high doses. Therefore, they should be used cautiously, particularly in elderly patients who are more susceptible.

Caregivers and family members need to be vigilant. If they observe any abnormal behavior, they must discuss it with a healthcare professional immediately. When prescribed dopamine agonists, the initial dose is typically small to prevent side effects. The dosage is then gradually increased over a few weeks, with anti-sickness medication prescribed if nausea becomes an issue. While a rare complication, sudden onset of sleep may occur during dopamine agonist therapy, so it is advisable to avoid driving while the dose is being increased.

Anticholinergics

Anticholinergics like benztropine (Cogentin) and trihexyphenidyl (Artane) are medications that help restore the balance between dopamine and acetylcholine in the brain. This can provide relief from tremors and muscle stiffness commonly experienced by individuals with Parkinson's disease. However, these drugs often have side effects such as impaired memory, confusion, hallucinations, constipation, dry mouth, and difficulty urinating. While they offer modest benefits, it's important to consider the potential drawbacks associated with their use.

MAO-B inhibitors

Safinamide (Xadago), selegiline (Eldepryl, Zelapar), and rasagiline are medications that block the breakdown of dopamine in the brain by inhibiting the brain enzyme monoamine oxidase B (MAO B). This enzyme breaks down brain dopamine. By doing so, they help increase the availability of dopamine, contributing to improved brain function.

Selegiline has shown some evidence of slowing the progression of Parkinson's disease, particularly in the early stages. However, it may cause common side effects such as nausea, dizziness, fainting, and stomach pain.

Similarly, animal studies suggest that rasagiline may also have a positive effect on slowing down the progression of Parkinson's disease. Its side effects may include headache, joint pain, indigestion, and depression.

Safinamide is an additional medication that may be prescribed to individuals already taking levodopa and carbidopa but are experiencing breakthrough Parkinson's symptoms. Studies have shown that adding safinamide can extend the duration of reduced or symptom-free periods. The most common side effects associated with safinamide include difficulty falling or staying asleep, nausea, falls, and uncontrolled involuntary movements.

It is important to note that when combined with carbidopa-levodopa, these medications may increase the risk of hallucinations. Moreover, MAO B inhibitors are generally not recommended to be taken simultaneously with most antidepressants or certain pain medications due to the potential for serious but rare reactions. It is advised to consult with your healthcare team before taking any additional medications with an MAO B inhibitor.

COMT inhibitors

COMT inhibitors, such as entacapone (Comtan), opicapone (Ongentys), and tolcapone (Tasmar), are medications that play a vital role in the treatment of Parkinson's disease. When levodopa, a key component for managing the symptoms, is taken, a chemical called COMT interferes with its efficacy by rendering a portion of the drug ineffective. However, the use of COMT inhibitors effectively blocks the action of COMT, allowing the brain to utilize levodopa more efficiently, ultimately relieving the symptoms associated with Parkinson's disease. Side effects include an increased risk of involuntary movements called dyskinesia, mainly resulting from an enhanced levodopa effect. Other side effects include diarrhea, nausea, or vomiting.

All of these medications are important components of Parkinson's disease treatment protocol. Still, it is essential to remember that the side effects associated with them must be discussed and monitored carefully. It is essential to work closely with your doctor when deciding which medications to take for Parkinson's disease, as different drugs will work differently for different people. Your healthcare provider can help you develop a personalized treatment plan that works best for you and your specific needs.

Dosage and Timing Considerations

Dosing for PD medications can be a tricky business, which is why a lot of emphasis is on understanding the interactions between drugs and their side effects. Taking the right amount of medicine at the right time is essential to maximize its effectiveness. It's also important to follow your doctor or pharmacist's instructions regarding when and how to take your medication. For example, some medicines may need to be taken with food, while others should be taken on an empty stomach. Additionally, some PD medications must be taken multiple times a day, while others can last up to 24 hours.

When it comes to taking your Parkinson's medications, timing is essential. The schedule isn't as simple as morning, noon, and night. There's a specific window during which you need to take your medications to maintain a steady dopamine level. Missing a dose can lead to "off periods," where you might feel the effects of the disease more intensely. It's important to establish a routine and consider using alarms or pill packs to stay on track.

I found that keeping a log of the medications taken was a big help. I would log the date, medication, amount, and the time it was taken. I used my iPhone timer to alert me to each new dosage time and recorded any noticeable reactions to the medication, such as increased dyskinesia, etc. It provided peace of mind and clarity for both my wife and myself and gave the doctor a diary of sorts to track the effectiveness of the treatment. Some people experience off periods as their disease progresses, so maintaining a consistent medication schedule becomes increasingly crucial. Forgetting a dose or delaying it can lead to shaky or unsteady feelings. Setting alarms or using pill packs can help prevent these situations.

It's worth noting that Parkinson's medications differ from over-the-counter drugs like Advil. They can have significant effects on your body, and adjusting the dosage should always be discussed with your doctor. Proper titration, either increasing or decreasing the dosage gradually, is essential to minimize side effects and ensure the medication's effectiveness.

When complications arise, particularly in the context of Parkinson's disease treatment, important decisions need to be made. Here's a breakdown of the situation and the available options:

If you notice symptoms re-emerging, this may indicate a phenomenon known as "off." At this juncture, two main approaches can be considered:

Increasing Levodopa Doses: One option is to increase the number of levodopa administrations to four, five, or even more times a day. However, it's crucial to recognize that increasing the frequency of levodopa intake can lead to poor adherence and become a complex regimen for patients to manage.

Using Adjunctive Medications: Another approach is to avoid continually increasing levodopa doses and instead consider using adjunctive medications. These drugs are designed to extend the effects of the existing levodopa tablets. Notably, medications like the COMT inhibitor or picabotine meet this criteria. These drugs can be taken once a day and effectively prolong the efficacy of individual levodopa doses.

A survey conducted among general neurologists and movement disorder specialists revealed insights into their approaches. Around 70-80% of specialists indicated that they would increase the levodopa intake. However, this might not be the best choice for patient outcomes due to the challenges associated with adherence and complex treatment regimens. Instead, an alternative proposal is to explore the use of drugs that can extend the effects of levodopa. One such example is the COMT inhibitor or picabotine, which requires only once-a-day dosing and offers an extension in the effectiveness of each levodopa dose.

Fortunately, medical advancements have led to the approval of alternative options for individuals experiencing OFF periods. For instance, an inhalable powder form of levodopa called INBRIJA has been developed to provide fast-acting relief during these periods. Additionally, the tablet istradefylline, marketed as Nourianz, has also been approved to address OFF periods. While increasing levodopa doses might appear more straightforward from a medical perspective, considering options that enhance the effects of existing levodopa doses can provide better outcomes and improved quality of life for patients. The goal is to optimize treatment strategies while ensuring that patients can manage their regimens effectively.

When it comes to optimizing your medication regimen, it's important to keep track of medication times meal times, and observe symptom patterns. Jotting down when your medication kicks in and wears off can help you visualize your needs. Remember to monitor any dyskinesias and note any side effects. As we have said, this record will be helpful during conversations with your specialist so that you can fine-tune your regimen for better symptom management.

Medication Guidelines for Parkinson's Disease

1. When starting new medications, discussing the potential side effects with your doctor and following your doctor's instructions regarding pill division or capsule separation is important. Even if you're feeling well, continuing your medication as prescribed is crucial to avoid worsening symptoms.

2. Always inform your doctor about any other medications you're taking, including over-the-counter drugs, herbal supplements, vitamins, and minerals.

3. Staying hydrated by drinking six to ten glasses of water daily is also recommended.

4. Establishing a consistent medication routine is key, so consider setting an alarm to remind yourself to take your medications at the same time each day. Familiarize yourself with your medications' names, doses, and possible side effects, and always carry a list of this information with you. Keep a medication calendar to track each amount you take.

5. If you miss a dose at your scheduled time, don't panic. Take it as soon as you remember. However, if it's almost time for your next dose, skip the missed dose and return to your regular medication schedule.

6. Remember, it's important not to keep outdated drugs. Get rid of them by following the instructions on the drug label or patient information sheet. Alternatively, you can check with your pharmacist about how to dispose of them. When storing drugs, ensure they are kept in a dry area away from moisture, unless your doctor or pharmacist tells you otherwise.

7. Don't share your medications with others. It's always a good idea to take extra medicine with you when you travel, in case you need to stay away longer than planned. Keep it in your carry-on luggage, not in a checked bag.

8. Lastly, refill your prescriptions before you completely run out of medicine. Give the pharmacy a call at least 48 hours before you run out. If you encounter difficulties in getting to the pharmacy, have financial concerns, or face any other obstacles that make it hard for you to get your medications, be sure to let your doctor know.

Remember, PD is a long journey and it is not always easy to stay ahead of your medication regimen. But if you take the right steps to make sure you are prepared, it can make all the difference.

In the next chapter, we are going to discuss the current technologies that can make your life easier and allow you to adapt to your new reality.

Chapter 5: Assistive Devices and Technology Guide for Parkinson's Patients and Caregivers

"My uncle told me that he had stopped drinking coffee or tea in public out of embarrassment. That's when I designed the no-spill cup. It functions purely based on its form. The curve on top deflects the liquid back inside every time they experience tremors, which keeps the liquid from spilling, unlike a normal cup. So, with one problem solved, there are still many more challenges to address." - Mileha Soneji, designer of low-tech tools for Parkinson's patients.

Having the freedom to stay active and independent as you go about your life is a privilege. A privilege that people with Parkinson's may not always have. When a diagnosis of Parkinson's is made, people usually imagine themselves in a wheelchair, unable to perform many of the activities they once did. And as the disease progresses, you can feel that freedom slipping away. It starts with decreased mobility, then fatigue and pain, followed by a more limited ability to move around and do everyday tasks.

Life becomes incredibly challenging in a world where one cannot speak, work, or move freely. The toll on mental health cannot be overlooked. The absence of autonomy and exclusion from society have a profound impact, resulting in depression and social isolation. But despite all of this, hope is still alive for people living with Parkinson's disease. With the help of assistive technology and devices, you can continue living your life as independently as possible. The global need for assistive technology is

51

staggering, with approximately 2.5 billion people, or roughly one-third of the world's population, requiring some form of assistive technology to enhance their lives. By using these tools, people with Parkinson's can remain active and mobile despite their disease.

In this chapter, we will provide an overview of available technologies for people with Parkinson's, discuss how they can be used to enhance mobility and independence and provide guidance on selecting assistive technology that is right for you. The goal of this chapter is to empower people living with Parkinson's to use technology in a way that helps them regain independence, increase mobility, and have a better quality of life.

Enhancing Mobility with Assistive Devices

A range of assistive devices exists to aid individuals with walking difficulties due to Parkinson's disease. These devices offer varying degrees of support tailored to individual needs and preferences. Choosing the right assistive device depends on your specific requirements at any given time. It's important to note that assistive devices for Parkinson's differ from those used for traditional orthopedic injuries. While orthopedic devices often alleviate weight-bearing, devices for Parkinson's primarily focus on enhancing balance.

The Single Point Cane is a super simple and budget-friendly solution that gives you that extra stability and support when you're out and about. With just one point of contact with the ground, it keeps you steady and works great for people who need a little help with balance. And the best part? It's totally portable, perfect for everyday use.

The Quad Cane is great because it provides enhanced stability and support with four contact points on the ground. This makes it super helpful for people dealing with balance challenges. It might feel a little awkward to manage compared to a regular cane, but the wider base gives you even more stability. Overall, the Quad Cane is a valuable aid for those needing added balance and support.

The Two-Wheel Walker is designed with two wheels on the front legs, offering stability and support. Although it can be challenging to maneuver, particularly in outdoor or crowded areas, it is an ideal choice for individuals with balance issues who require more support than a cane.

The Four-Wheel Walker is designed to provide stability and ease of maneuverability. Equipped with four wheels, it may also include a seat for resting. This walker offers support for walking and is particularly useful for longer distances. It is important to note that the seat should not be used while the walker is in motion.

Wheelchairs and power chairs are for individuals who have difficulty walking for extended periods. These mobility aids provide support, stability, and the ability to travel longer distances easily. Wheelchairs may be manual or powered, depending on an individual's needs. Power chairs offer even more independence, allowing users to get around independently without relying on another person for assistance.

Proper training on how to effectively and safely use the chosen mobility aid is absolutely essential for individuals seeking to enhance their mobility and make the most out of its numerous benefits. By providing comprehensive guidance and instruction, individuals can ensure their personal safety and optimize the advantages offered by the mobility aid they have selected. This training equips users with the necessary knowledge and techniques to navigate their surroundings confidently, leading to increased independence and improved overall quality of life.

Communication Aids for Parkinson's Patients

Speech and voice changes are prevalent among individuals with Parkinson's disease, affecting approximately 90% of those diagnosed. These changes go beyond mere slowness or muscle rigidity; they are attributed to an internal scheduling issue in the brain, often referred to as a scaling problem. This problem makes it challenging for individuals with Parkinson's to regulate the loudness of their voice or the movements of their tongue and jaw necessary for clear speech.

The range of speech changes in Parkinson's includes a decreased vocal volume, resulting in a quieter voice than before. Some may develop a breathy or hoarse quality to their voice. The speech rate can be affected, with some experiencing a slowing down of speech while others exhibit an increased speech rate. In a small percentage of cases (6-13%), very fast speech rates, known as "tachyphemia," can develop, causing speech sounds to become jumbled and resembling the speech patterns seen in individuals with stuttering. Although the content may be accurate, the process of articulating their thoughts might take longer. This delay in idea formulation can result in impaired turn-taking, as extended pauses disrupt the natural flow of conversation. This can leave conversation partners wondering when it's their turn to contribute.

Individuals with Parkinson's may also face challenges in using gestures effectively. Gestures can support verbal communication, but reduced gesture usage further complicates the dynamics of conversation for those with Parkinson's.

When addressing communication disorders in Parkinson's, a cookbook or one-size-fits-all approach is inadequate. Effective intervention demands a diverse toolkit with multiple tools, strategies, and approaches to optimize communication in various settings.

Exercise is a vital component of this toolkit, and the **Lee Silverman Voice Treatment (LSVT)** stands out as a well-researched program. Developed by Laurie Ramig and Cynthia Fox, LSVT is an intensive exercise regimen targeting voice loudness, articulation, speech clarity, and facial expression. This systematic approach recalibrates the loudness and effort needed for communication, benefitting many individuals. However, it might not be suitable for those with advanced disease or significant cognitive changes.

Expanding beyond LSVT, a new approach involves **Expiratory Muscle Strength Training (EMST),** focusing on respiratory support for speech. Developed by Christine Sapienza's team, EMST enhances speech volume and may impact swallowing. Using a specialized device, this at-home program lasts around four weeks and requires daily 30-minute sessions.

Additionally, an intriguing natural phenomenon, the Lombard effect, comes into play. This effect prompts individuals to raise their voice volume in noisy environments. Interestingly, the Lombard effect remains functional in Parkinson's, providing an avenue for therapy optimization. To optimize the Lombard effect and enhance voice volume in individuals with Parkinson's, various therapy approaches and devices have been developed. One such device is the **Speech 5**, designed by Jessica Huber and her team. This small device, similar to a hearing aid, is worn in the ear. When the individual starts speaking, the device introduces background noise simulating a crowded environment. This encourages the individual to naturally raise their voice volume without conscious effort, making it particularly helpful for those with cognitive challenges.

Another innovative approach involves the **"iParkinsons" iPhone app**. This app uses the phone's microphone to monitor the loudness of the individual's voice. When the voice volume drops below a certain level, the app delivers multi-talker background noise to the individual's ear, prompting them to adjust their voice volume higher. This again harnesses the Lombard effect to enhance communication.

For individuals struggling with excessive speech rate, which affects about 6 to 13 percent of people with Parkinson's, **delayed auditory feedback (DAF) devices** offer a solution. These devices play back the individual's speech at a slight delay, leading to a natural reduction in speech rate. This method is effective and can significantly improve speech intelligibility.

Pacing boards are another technique to address rapid speech rate. These boards consist of marked targets, such as circles or crosses, corresponding to each word. When the individual touches a target while speaking each word, it automatically slows down their speech rate. Pacing boards offer a quick and portable solution to manage excessive speech rates.

Voice amplifiers are portable devices that pick up the user's voice and project it at a higher volume, making it easier for others to hear. These devices can be especially beneficial for individuals with Parkinson's who struggle to produce a sufficiently loud voice. Voice amplifiers can be worn discreetly around the waist or clipped to clothing. They come in various sizes and can be funded by insurance or support agencies. Some devices are specifically designed for telephone communication, amplifying incoming and outgoing voices.

Another approach uses **FM systems,** which involve a transmitter worn by the speaker (person with Parkinson's) and a receiver worn by the listener (conversation partner). This wireless system directly amplifies the speaker's voice and delivers it to the listener's ears, enhancing communication clarity. FM systems offer a more personalized and adaptable solution, allowing multiple listeners to adjust their own volume levels and enabling better communication between rooms. These systems can also be set up in larger spaces, such as meeting rooms, using loop systems for broader coverage.

The combination of exercise programs, therapy approaches, and communication devices, such as voice amplifiers and FM systems, forms a multi-faceted strategy for improving communication for individuals with Parkinson's disease. These tools aim to reduce communication effort, enhance speech clarity, and promote effective interactions between individuals with Parkinson's and their conversation partners. The overall focus is on adapting communication methods and engaging in proactive strategies to navigate cognitive and vocal challenges associated with Parkinson's disease. Establishing a supportive network of loved ones and healthcare professionals is important to enhance communication and overall well-being.

Adaptive Equipment for Daily Activities

In the journey towards managing Parkinson's disease, individuals and their caregivers are presented with a multitude of challenges that can impact their daily routines and overall quality of life. As the condition progresses, even simple activities that were once taken for granted can become increasingly difficult to perform independently. However, adaptive equipment can help to provide an effective solution for maintaining independence.

Eating

These assistive devices can be beneficial for individuals with Parkinson's disease or other conditions that affect grip strength, dexterity, and tremors. These devices are designed to make daily tasks like eating and drinking more manageable. Here's a rundown of each device mentioned:

1. Weighted Cutlery can be helpful for individuals with tremors, as it provides added weight to utensils to help stabilize hand movements during eating. Not everyone may benefit, so trying before purchasing is recommended.

2. Smart Technology, such as the Liftware Spoon, utilizes advanced features to stabilize utensils and counteract the effects of shaky hands or tremors. This innovation helps individuals with motor impairments maintain control and independence in their daily lives.

3. Assive utensils like the Built-Up Utensil have been designed to cater to individuals with reduced grip strength. These utensils feature a larger handle that is easier to hold onto, ensuring a more comfortable dining experience.

4. Another option is the Universal Cup, which benefits individuals with limited grip and dexterity. This versatile cup can also be used with other items like toothbrushes or razors. It provides a more secure grip for holding and drinking from a cup.

5. To prevent mealtime mishaps, the Plate Guard is easily attachable and detachable from round plates. It effectively prevents food from being pushed off the plate while also offering a stable surface for scooping food.

6. For those who struggle with tremors or weakness while drinking, the Spillproof Cup with Handles proves to be a valuable solution. The cup's design helps individuals maintain control, preventing spills, while the handles provide a more secure grip.

Together, these products provide a comprehensive solution to individuals with limited dexterity or grip. They offer an improved eating and drinking experience, helping users maintain their independence.

Devices for Meal Preparation

Meal preparation and cooking tasks can be challenging for individuals with Parkinson's disease or limited hand function. However, specialized adaptive tools are available to make these tasks more manageable. Let's take a look at some of these tools:

1. One such tool is the adapted cutting board. This cutting board has spikes that hold the food in place, allowing individuals to focus on cutting with one hand. It is particularly helpful for those who struggle with coordination using both hands. Additionally, plastic supports on the board assist with cutting and buttering tasks.
2. Another helpful tool is the rocker knife. This knife is designed to reduce pain and the risk of injury while cutting. It features a T-shaped handle for easy grip, enabling cutting with a rocking motion and applying less pressure.
3. For individuals with reduced hand function, the palm peeler comes in handy. This tool fits in the palm of the hand and is used to easily peel fruits and vegetables by running the hand over them.
4. Dyson non-slip material is used to keep items like cutting boards, graters, or mixing bowls secure on the table. This high-grip material prevents slipping and provides stability during kitchen tasks.

These adaptive tools offer significant benefits, enhancing kitchen tasks for individuals facing specific challenges. They promote independence and make daily activities more accessible. Occupational therapists can provide personalized recommendations and training on effectively using these tools based on individual needs. By incorporating assistive devices into meal preparation, individuals can overcome obstacles and enjoy the benefits of independent and efficient cooking.

Assistive Devices for Dressing

Privacy and autonomy are key components of successful living for individuals with physical limitations. Assistive dressing devices provide an independent means to get dressed. One such device is the button hook, which is particularly useful for those with fine motor control or grip challenges. By inserting the device through the buttonhole and looping it around the button, individuals can effortlessly fasten their buttons.

Another helpful device is the zipper pull, designed for individuals who struggle with gripping small zipper tabs. With a loop that allows the use of the thumb or finger, the zipper can be easily pulled up or down, making it more accessible for everyone.

The dressing stick comes in handy for individuals with limited mobility in the shoulder or hip or limited grip strength. This device aids in putting on or taking off clothing items, thanks to its vinyl-coated stick that easily grips onto clothing.

In addition, the sock aid is designed for putting on socks without needing to bend at the hip. By placing the sock onto a tube and inserting the foot into the tube, the handles can be pulled to effortlessly slide the sock on.

Occupational therapists play a crucial role in guiding individuals in selecting and effectively using these devices based on their specific needs and challenges. Their expertise ensures that individuals receive the necessary support and guidance to maximize the benefits of these assistive devices.

Assistive Technology for Home Safety

While independence and freedom are essential to maintaining morale, coming up with a home safety plan is also crucial in ensuring that the individual remains safe and secure. Home safety involves ensuring the physical environment is free from potential hazards, such as having good lighting, removing rugs and clutter, and using non-slip mats.

For PD patients, using assistive technology resources such as accessible door locks, alert systems for falls, and remote health monitoring systems can help maintain a safe home environment. Occupational therapists can advise and guide in assessing the individual's needs and selecting the most suitable assistive devices to ensure their safety at home. In addition, they can also suggest adaptations that may be necessary, such as re-arranging furniture and simplifying tasks. People with Parkinson's should also be aware of potential dangers in the home that could lead to falls or other accidents, such as loose wires, boxes, or clutter on the floor.

Additionally, installing safety items such as grab bars near toilets and showers can help prevent falls. Here are some of the assistive devices used often:

1. Transfer Boards: Used to help transfer from a seated position to another surface.
2. Hospital Beds: Allow for position changes and aid with various health conditions.
3. Bed Rails: Prevent falling out of bed and assist with repositioning.
4. Standing Grab Bars: Provide stability and aid in sit-to-stand transitions.
5. Bed Ladders: Help individuals sit up in bed when it's difficult.
6. Blanket Cradles: Keep blankets off the feet and assist with movement.

Ultimately, the focus should be to provide solutions, not create further problems by ignoring safety and chasing freedom. Caregivers are the first line of defense when it comes to assisting a loved one. They are knowledgeable about the needs and capabilities of their patients, so they should be in the loop when selecting the right assistive devices that will help them remain safe and independent. With the right tools and guidance, you can not only survive but thrive.

In the next chapter, we will discuss the mental health impact of Parkinson's on both the caregiver and the patient.

Chapter 6: Emotional Support and Mental Health Guide for Parkinson's Patients and Caregivers

"I was told, "Jimmy, you have Parkinson's." It all started with stiffness, rigidity, and, at times, loss of balance. But I found myself months later, sitting in my neurologist's office, head down in disbelief. "Parkinson's? Are you kidding me? This is a disease for old people, right? I'm young. This can't be true. I don't believe it. In fact, that's how I treated it. I was going to ignore it, and it was going to go away. Out of mind, out of sight. Give me the blue pill, right Morpheus? Put me back in the matrix. But fortunately, that's not how things work." - Jimmy Choi, a member of The Michael J. Fox Foundation (MJFF) Patient Council, diagnosed with young-onset Parkinson's disease at age 27.

Parkinson's diagnosis is a moment of stillness amidst a whirlwind of emotions. Uncertainties, hopes, and fears collide, weighed down by the unfairness of fate. Time becomes a concept both distant and imminent. A million questions surge in your mind.

Why me?

Why now?

How long do I have?

Am I going to be able to keep living my life?

No one plans for this to happen. Nor do we expect this to happen to our loved ones. And while you are still in the whirlpool of all the emotional impact, you have disease progression to worry about. The medication, your job, your relationship, your children. How do you navigate this new terrain?

Taking care of your emotional well-being is just as crucial to your physical health as exercise and medications when it comes to living with PD. A diagnosis of Parkinson's, along with the constantly evolving symptoms that come with its progression, can trigger an array of emotions for both you and your loved ones. All your plans for the future are put on hold, and all the "what ifs" take over your thoughts. So, let's try to work through these emotions and learn to cope with them.

Understanding the Emotional Impact of Parkinson's Disease

The emotional impact of Parkinson's is vast and unique to each individual. Just as any regular person who gets devastating news, your first and instinctual response is going to be denial. Denial is the way our mind protects itself from shock. It's also a way for us to take time and adjust to the changes that come with this new diagnosis. You have got the answer, but it isn't what you wanted, so you are trying to make sense of it.

Fear is another emotion that follows in the wake of a Parkinson's diagnosis. You are frightened about what this will mean for your future and how others will perceive you. It can be incredibly daunting when you think of all the treatment uncertainty that comes with living with the disease.

Anger and frustration can also creep in. You may feel frustrated that no one can give you a definitive answer as to what treatment will be best for you or how your life will look in ten years. Anger may even be directed towards those who don't understand your condition or yourself for being diagnosed with it.

Sadness is a natural response to being diagnosed with Parkinson's as you come to terms with the reality of the situation. You may feel overwhelmed by how much your life will change or regret that you can no longer do things that used to give you pleasure. It can be hard to accept that life isn't going to pan out the way you planned, but it is important to remember that although Parkinson's can have a significant impact on your life, it doesn't mean you can't still find joy and fulfillment. So, how do you fix the way you feel?

The answer is complex and challenging. You cannot just flip a switch and move forward to the next phase of emotional response. It's important to remember that all these emotions are normal and valid. Even though it may be hard to process them, you must allow yourself to feel these emotions to move forward with your treatment plan and live a full life. You must take the time to process your feelings and find ways to cope. That can be done in a variety of ways.

Coping Strategies for Patients

The shift in your reality can be pretty overwhelming. It's important to find healthy ways to cope with this new reality and take care of yourself. The internet is ripe with all the tips and tricks you can do to cope with the diagnosis of PD. But here's the thing. You are not supposed to be just coping with PD; you are also supposed to be living. Living with PD may mean that things have changed and that it's natural to feel fear or anxiety at times. But it doesn't mean you can't still have moments of joy, hope, and love. It's essential to find ways to enjoy life, and you can use some of Emma Lawton's tricks, who was diagnosed with PD at 27, to get there.

Be open and honest about what is going on with you. It's okay to say you are having a bad day. It's okay to not be okay. If you experience the worst of days, then you will experience the best of days. You have to feel that unhappiness to feel the happiness that you get from a good day and from good things happening in your life. By being honest with others, you help them understand how to treat you, what you expect from them, and when and where you need assistance. It simplifies things for all because every time you share about your Parkinson's, you know it tugs at their heartstrings. Even if it's the tenth time you've mentioned it, it's the first time they're hearing it.

Appreciate the small things: Don't sweat the small stuff, but appreciate the small things you can do. So, don't get hung up on the day-to-day little things if you can, but enjoy the things that you may usually take for granted. Focus on what you can control. Taking control of situations when possible will help you minimize stress. Every day is a new beginning, and every morning, you have the potential to start anew.

By **acknowledging your challenges**, you can take back control and work through them. You may not know why these things are happening, but it's important to accept them and figure out ways of dealing with them. This could be as simple as accepting that some days will be harder than others and taking the time to practice self-care.

Be impatient with yourself, not with other people. Be impatient with yourself, and don't settle. You could have very easily hidden in a corner, doing nothing for the rest of your life, and no one would have judged you for it because it's a big thing to deal with. But you do more now than you've ever done before, and that's because you feel like you have nothing to lose. Live as if it's the last opportunity to do something. Say yes more.

Lastly, **be kind**. Remember that everyone is going through something as well. It might be something tiny to you, but it might be something massive to them. Being kind to others and realizing that everyone's road is different can be what helps get you through. Recognize that it's okay to take time for yourself and ensure you're taking care of yourself. Ultimately, self-care is the best way to make sure that you stay healthy mentally and physically. By being more tolerant of others, it makes you happier in yourself.

Coping Strategies for Caregivers

As a caregiver of someone with Parkinson's disease, you have taken on a challenging and multifaceted role. You help maintain your loved one's quality of life while educating yourself about the disease's symptoms, treatments, and progression. You also diligently track doctor's appointments, medication schedules, and exercise routines. Above all, you provide the love and support necessary to navigate the challenges of Parkinson's disease. Being a caregiver is undoubtedly challenging, but your dedication and compassion make a significant difference in your loved one's life. I know firsthand that the amount of tasks can be overwhelming, and the worry for one's charge can be draining. Here are a few coping strategies for caretakers to make the experience easier:

1. You cannot pour from an empty cup, so take time for yourself. Make sure you have time to relax and recharge, ultimately making you a better caregiver. If needed, seek support from family members or consider hiring assistance to help with caregiving responsibilities. This was a lesson I had to learn the hard way, as they say on every flight. "If the oxygen masks drop down, put on your mask first and then help someone else."
2. Knowledge is power, so learn as much as you can about your loved one's disease. By doing so, you will gain insight into the potential behavioral or symptomatic alterations your loved one might experience and learn how you can offer the most effective assistance during these occurrences.
3. Let your loved one take part. Don't feel like you have to do everything for them. Give them the space and time to handle daily tasks themselves, like getting dressed.

4. Make sure to have a heartfelt conversation with your loved ones about their family affairs. Although it may not be the easiest topic to discuss, knowing their wishes regarding a living will, durable power of attorney, and do-not-resuscitate (DNR) order is important.

5. Make sure to set realistic goals for yourself and your loved one. Don't try to do everything. By setting goals that are within reach, you're setting everyone up for success instead of disappointment.

6. Don't put your life on hold! Keep meeting with friends, doing hobbies or joining groups, and maintaining your regular schedule. I know it can be hard, but trust me, you'll feel more energized and less likely to feel resentful.

7. Having open and honest communication about expectations is a must. Speak openly, and be sure to listen to your loved one's needs. Be open to compromise when it's necessary and express gratitude for their help in managing caregiving tasks.

8. Try to forgive yourself when you can't do everything. Feeling guilty for not being able to do it all is common, but remember that you are doing the best you can. Don't forget to look after yourself too. In my case, as time progressed, occasionally, I would get a little impatient. She would notice, stop, and look at me with frustration in her eyes. I felt terrible and would say, "I'm sorry, I forgot." Sometimes, you may have to ask for forgiveness, too.

9. Finally, make sure you have someone you can confide in. Along with offering a listening ear and support to your loved ones, it's helpful to have someone who can be there for you, too. Openly and honestly share your feelings with a friend or family member. If that's not feasible, consider joining a support group. Realizing that you're not alone and that others are going through similar experiences can provide a sense of comfort.

Professional Counseling and Therapy Options

Deciding to seek counseling is a crucial step. Many times, people don't reach out for help due to feelings of guilt, shame, or embarrassment. But by choosing to get help, you've made a choice to feel better and improve your life. It's important to select counseling services carefully, ensuring they meet your needs. Working with a trained mental health care provider and your doctor will help you create the right treatment plan.

First, you and your doctor should review how you and those around you are handling your illness. It's crucial to understand that Parkinson's disease can have a significant impact on your mental well-being, alongside the physical symptoms and challenges. The changes happening in your brain can sometimes lead to depression, which is as real a part of the disease as tremors or slowed movement.

Sometimes, medical treatment for depression may be necessary. So, if you're feeling down, your doctor might suggest you see a mental health specialist for an assessment. These specialists can include family therapists, social workers, psychologists, psychiatrists, or other professionals. They'll be able to provide valuable insights and support for your mental health.

Types of Counseling

The following list briefly describes common types of counseling. These can be used together or alone, depending on your treatment plan.

Crisis intervention counseling: When you find yourself in a crisis, like feeling overwhelmed by a diagnosis, crisis intervention counseling steps in to assist you. The counselor will support you during this difficult time and, if necessary, guide you toward additional counseling or medical care. You can access these services through community health agencies, helplines, and hotlines.

Individual counseling is when you have one-on-one sessions with a counselor. It usually happens in the privacy of their office. This type of counseling is effective when your problems stem from your own thoughts and behaviors. It's also beneficial for personal issues that are hard to discuss in a group setting. If you're dealing with depression, anxiety, or grief related to Parkinson's, this kind of counseling might be right for you.

Family therapy can be beneficial in dealing with Parkinson's disease. It affects the whole family. If you're the primary breadwinner, it can put a strain on your finances. And if you're the one taking care of the house, you might have to change how chores are divided. These everyday challenges and the emotional toll of dealing with a chronic illness really shake up the family dynamic.

Family therapy is a great way to resolve issues among family members and help them support each other better. It might involve the whole family or just a few members. The therapist will work with you to find ways to talk about and manage the challenging aspects of living with Parkinson's, like social isolation, fatigue, and changes in mobility. There are also techniques for helping those affected by Parkinson's get better sleep and focus on maintaining their physical health.

Group therapy. In group therapy, you join a group to talk about problems together. You've got a counselor who sort of guides the session. Those in the group usually have similar issues, but sometimes they don't. The best thing about these group sessions is that it's a safe place where you can open up to others who get what you're going through. It's a chance to learn about yourself and how others perceive you, too.

Residential treatment involves residing at a treatment center. The duration of the stay may vary depending on the program and therapy progress, ranging from a few weeks to over a year. These programs are available in various settings, such as hospitals, home-like structures, and clinics.

Although all of the different types of therapies are available to help you through the grim times, they can only be utilized if you are open and honest about your emotions and feelings. Being able to talk about them can be difficult at first, but the more you open up, the easier it will get over time. It's important to remember that therapy is not an overnight solution; it takes time and dedication for results to occur. But if you persist, eventually, you'll see positive changes in yourself and learn how to cope with life's struggles.

Support Groups and Online Communities

There are more than 10 million people living with Parkinson's worldwide, and many of them feel the same way. It's a trying time that can be hard to navigate alone. But you're not alone. There are countless resources available to help you understand your diagnosis, manage symptoms, and live a full life with Parkinson's. Educating yourself about the disease is the first step in regaining control of your future. Networking with other patients can be invaluable in understanding how to cope and gaining access to support systems that will help you along the way.

Support groups and online communities are great resources for those with Parkinson's and their families. Whether online or in-person, these support networks will allow you to meet other patients who understand what you're going through, as well as family members who have loved ones living with the disease. Many of these groups also offer educational programs, recreation activities, and other beneficial resources.

Here are some well-known support groups and organizations that can help you find the support you need:

The Parkinson's Foundation

American Parkinson Disease Association (APDA)

Michael J. Fox Foundation for Parkinson's Research

PatientsLikeMe

Parkinson's Movement Disorder and Alliance (PMD Alliance)

NeuroTalk

These organizations are committed to providing resources, education, and support for individuals living with Parkinson's disease and their families. They offer access to clinical trials, disease-specific programs, online forums, webinars, and more. With their help, you can gain the information and support necessary for navigating life with Parkinson's. The best part is, you don't have to go it alone. There are people out there who understand what you're going through and can provide information, resources, and emotional support – all for free. So explore the offerings of these organizations and get the help you need to live a better life with Parkinson's disease.

You can also check out other online resources, such as blogs and websites dedicated to Parkinson's. These are excellent resources of current information about the disease and its treatments, as well as personal stories from people living with the condition. They can help provide a sense of community and understanding that is helpful when dealing with a chronic illness.

Finally, don't forget to reach out to your local Parkinson's organizations. Many of these have support groups and educational programs that can help you stay informed, connected, and inspired. And if you don't find what you need there, they can often point you in the right direction. No matter how overwhelming it may seem at times, living with Parkinson's disease doesn't have to be a lonely or isolating experience. With the right information and support network, you can thrive in spite of this condition.

In the next chapter, we will review the tips for sleep management and how to get the best rest while living with Parkinson's. By practicing these methods, you can improve your overall quality of life and well-being. Stay tuned!

Chapter 7: Sleep and Fatigue Management Guide for Parkinson's Patients and Caregivers

"Anybody with Parkinson's will tell you that when you go to sleep, you know you can start the night with the best intentions, and I always have done. You try your best to get to sleep. I can't remember the last time I slept through. Yeah, every night's broken dreams, broken sleep, because the stiffness wakes us up, the rigidity, and with the best will in the world, I would wake up at half past two, three, four, and you know, last night was horrible. It was one of the longest nights. I hope I sleep better tonight." –

Anonymous

People often talk about how PD acts by attacking your body, mind, and spirit. It affects your daily life, including your sleep. Imagine trying to get your body ready for a night of rest, but instead, you are dealing with stiffness, rigidity, and difficulty moving. It's no wonder why many people living with PD wake up multiple times during the night.

We spend about a third of our lives sleeping. There is strong evidence suggesting that the quality of our sleep can have a direct impact on various aspects of our lives. For instance, studies indicate that good sleep can improve memory, enhance thinking and concentration, boost mood and overall well-being, and prevent daytime sleepiness. Furthermore, adequate sleep increases energy and improves physical performance.

Why Sleep Is Important

Sleep is crucial for both brain and body functioning. It impacts our mood, cognitive abilities (such as thinking and creativity), judgment, attention, and concentration. Additionally, sleep plays a vital role in our body's restorative functions, including immune system function and hormone regulation. It helps protect against infections, minimize the impact of stress, and regulate various bodily processes.

So, how much sleep should you get to ensure you are well-rested? Well, for individuals over 65, the target range is typically seven to eight hours. However, it's important to note that **sleep quantity** alone doesn't tell the whole story. The **quality** of your sleep is just as important to consider. You see, it's not enough to simply get eight hours of sleep if it's interrupted and fragmented throughout the night. In fact, you might find that you function best with a solid six hours of restful sleep. It may not sound like a lot, but having uninterrupted, high-quality sleep can make a world of difference. So, when discussing your sleep needs and assessing your sleep patterns, it's crucial to consider both the quality and quantity.

As we age, our sleep patterns naturally undergo changes. The duration of sleep tends to decrease, and its quality becomes lighter. This shift is characterized by a shorter period to fall asleep, an earlier bedtime, and waking up earlier in the morning. Moreover, sleep becomes more restless, resulting in increased episodes of awakening during the night. Bear in mind that these are just the natural changes with aging. This problem is further compounded for people with PD. Let's take a closer look at why.

Sleep Disorders Associated with Parkinson's Disease

Unfortunately, 66 to 80 percent of those with Parkinson's report that they have poor sleep quality. That's from a 2018 report from the Parkinson's Foundation. So, sleep is obviously a huge problem for people who have PD. The specific features of the condition can disrupt our sleep system. The degradation of sleep-regulating regions in the brain and dopaminergic centers directly affects our sleep, particularly REM sleep, as we will discuss in detail.

The disease symptoms also make a difference in your sleep. The **motor symptoms** like tremors, rigidity, and dystonia can make it difficult to sleep and be comfortable in a sleeping position. **Nocturia:** Waking up frequently to use the bathroom can also interrupt sleep. And then **psychiatric**

symptoms like depression, anxiety, or Parkinson 's-related hallucinations can interrupt your sleep.

We also know that there are **medication effects**. Medications that you might take specifically for Parkinson's can affect your sleep. So, really, anything that you're taking for Parkinson's can be disrupting your sleep or can be helping your sleep.

And another factor that I think is important is how **stressful** Parkinson's might be. We can all agree that stress and changes in your life will affect your sleep. Having Parkinson's disease and managing those symptoms, managing your appointments, managing your relationships with others, and continuing to lead a high quality of life can sometimes be very stressful. Any significant changes in life or big stressors in life can lead to sleep problems.

Finally, environmental factors like noise or light in the room can affect your ability to sleep as well. Let's go through specific sleep disorders and the problems that may manifest with these disorders. The first is what we call insomnia disorder.

Insomnia Disorder

Insomnia disorder is very straightforward—problems falling asleep, staying asleep, waking up too early in the morning, or some combination of all three. Insomnia disorder manifests as daytime fatigue or sleepiness during the day. It can also contribute to a poor mood, like an anxious or depressed mood. People with insomnia will also say they have difficulty with attention and memory. One way that many people with insomnia describe their day is that they feel *tired but wired*. You feel kind of in your bones that you are sleep-deprived; however, you couldn't go to sleep even if you wanted to. It's like feeling sleep-deprived but having your brain be too alert to go to sleep.

The treatment we have for insomnia disorder is called **Cognitive Behavioral Therapy for Insomnia (CBTI)**, which is a combination of cognitive behavioral therapy and lifestyle changes. CBTI helps people identify thoughts, beliefs, or behaviors contributing to insomnia and teaches them how to manage their sleep-wake schedule more effectively. This can involve learning relaxation techniques, improving sleep hygiene, and making changes like blocking out noise or avoiding caffeine in the afternoon.

CBTI also includes strategies to help people with insomnia challenge unhelpful thoughts that might be holding them back from getting quality sleep. It's important to note that it can take several weeks of consistent effort to reap the long-term rewards of CBTI. With a strong commitment to the program, people can experience improvements in sleep quality and an overall improvement in well-being.

There are other options for treating insomnia disorder, including sleep medications. What we know about medications for insomnia disorder is that even among relatively healthy people who do not have another chronic medical condition, sleep medications can be hit or miss. Sometimes they work well, sometimes they don't, and sometimes they work at first but lose effectiveness over time. As we get older, our body metabolizes these medications differently, which can lead to serious side effects like dizziness, problems with balance, and a greater risk of falling. So, medications for sleep may not be a great idea if you are having severe movement-related symptoms with your PD.

Sleep-Related Breathing Disorder

The second disorder that's very common in PD is called sleep-related breathing disorders. The two most common are **obstructive sleep apnea** and **central sleep apnea**. The prevalence rate for this is really high in PD, at about 20 to 60 percent of people with Parkinson's. Breathing disorders like sleep apnea are actually very common in the general population, too; anywhere from 10 to 15 percent of people have sleep apnea or some breathing disorder related to sleep. But of course, that prevalence rate is much higher in PD.

Sleep apnea is a condition where breathing is repeatedly interrupted during sleep. Essentially, you may hold your breath or not breathe optimally, sometimes accompanied by a decrease in blood oxygen levels. Consequently, your brain wakes up or becomes more alert to ensure proper breathing. Symptoms include fatigue, excessive sleepiness, possible morning headaches, and difficulties with attention and memory. Unlike individuals with insomnia, those with sleep-related breathing disorders are able to sleep during the day.

When it comes to sleep-related breathing disorders, the gold standard for treatment is the use of CPAP (Continuous Positive Airway Pressure) or BiPAP (Bi-level Positive Airway Pressure) machines. These devices provide continuous airflow to keep the airway open during sleep, ensuring proper oxygenation and preventing interruptions in breathing. However, if CPAP or BiPAP is not tolerable or suitable for you, there are alternative options available. One such option is using dental devices or mouthguards specifically designed to help keep your airway open. These custom-made devices can be created to fit your unique needs, providing an effective solution to improve your breathing during sleep. In some cases, airway surgeries may be recommended to open your airway further and alleviate the breathing difficulties associated with sleep-related disorders. These surgical procedures are tailored to address specific anatomical abnormalities that may contribute to airway obstruction.

It is important to consult with a healthcare professional specializing in sleep medicine to determine the most suitable treatment option for your condition. They can assess your individual needs and guide you toward the most appropriate intervention to ensure restful and uninterrupted sleep.

REM Sleep Behavior Disorder

When we dream, our brains generate various scenarios and activities, but to prevent us from physically acting out these dreams, a natural paralysis mechanism is in place. Many people might recall dreams where they're trying to shout or run, but their voice or legs don't respond. This is due to this paralysis during dreaming.

During sleep, we have different stages: light sleep, deep sleep, and REM sleep. Most of our night is light sleep, about 50%. 20 to 25% of your night is deep sleep, where body restoration happens. REM sleep, or Rapid Eye Movement sleep, is the other 20 to 25% of your sleep, and it's where brain restoration happens. Your brain is very active during REM sleep to do all the repair work it needs to do. During REM sleep, our body has learned to paralyze itself because we don't want to act out what we're experiencing in our brain during REM sleep, as it can be very vivid, strange, or even a nightmare activity.

However, in Parkinson's disease, the deterioration of the neural system responsible for maintaining this paralysis can occur. As a result, some individuals with PD may experience a situation where they physically enact the actions they're dreaming about. This is RBD or REM Sleep Behavior Disorder. To be clear, this isn't sleepwalking, as during these episodes, the person can't actually walk around. For example, if they're dreaming of delivering a lecture, they might start speaking as if they're giving that lecture. Alternatively, if they're dreaming of a physical altercation, they might move as if they're fighting.

Around half of all Parkinson's patients may encounter this phenomenon, and it's often one of the early signs of the disease. Interestingly, this can occur many years before other Parkinson's symptoms manifest, similar to losing the sense of smell. However, this can pose challenges for both the individual experiencing it and their sleeping partner. The main concern is the risk of injury, as someone might unintentionally harm themselves or their partner while enacting their dreams. First and foremost, we have to take safety precautions if someone has REM sleep behavior disorder to make sure that if they do act out their dreams, they won't harm themselves. To address the physical movements during sleep, here are some recommendations from a sleep physician:

1. If you're sleeping on a bed that's elevated around 2 feet off the ground, consider lowering it to prevent falls.
2. If you have a hospital-type bed with side rails, pad the rails to prevent injuries.
3. Pad the floor to ensure safety during movements.
4. Keep nightstands, large windows, and other potential hazards away from the bed.
5. Some individuals might need to sleep separately from their bed partners to prevent injuries.
6. In more severe cases, individuals might sleep in a sleeping bag to limit movement.
7. Medications can be used if the condition is bothersome. Melatonin is a commonly used hormone that can suppress dream-related behaviors. It's available over-the-counter and has minimal side effects, such as mild drowsiness.
8. Clonazepam (Klonopin) is another option that effectively slows down brain processing to suppress behaviors, but it can lead to drowsiness and increased fall risk, particularly in individuals with Parkinson's disease.
9. Lorazepam (Ativan) is a less-studied alternative with fewer side effects, but it might not be as effective as clonazepam.

The last two medications should only be used under the care of a healthcare provider.

Restless Leg Syndrome

Restless leg syndrome is a common condition that often accompanies sleep disorders. Interestingly, it is even more prevalent in individuals with Parkinson's disease. There are four main symptoms associated with restless leg syndrome.

People typically **experience sensations** like creepy crawlies or an unpleasant sand-like feeling in their legs. These sensations, although difficult to describe, originate from the brain rather than the legs themselves. The discomfort is usually heightened at night when lying down or resting.

Additionally, people often experience an **irresistible urge** to move their legs or stretch while trying to sleep. This can lead to **disturbed sleep** and fatigue during the day. **Movement** tends to alleviate the sensations, and they usually worsen in the evening.

Restless leg syndrome is not caused by a dopamine deficiency but rather by a difficulty in dopamine transportation in the brain. It is more prevalent in Parkinson's disease, possibly due to the use of medications that affect dopamine. Prolonged use of these drugs can exacerbate restless leg syndrome.

Diagnosis of restless leg syndrome relies on clinical evaluation as there isn't a specific test available. In some instances, restless leg syndrome may be accompanied by periodic limb movements during sleep, which are often linked to low iron levels. Iron is essential for dopamine transportation, and conditions like anemia or kidney disease can contribute to the development of restless leg syndrome.

When it comes to treatment, the first step is to figure out if intervention is necessary. There are certain medications, like some antidepressants and antihistamines, that can actually make the condition worse. On top of that, nicotine, caffeine, and alcohol have the potential to worsen symptoms too. If iron levels are low, taking supplements might help.

For more severe cases, there are prescription drugs available, such as gabapentin and pregabalin. Another option to consider is using dopamine agonist drugs like pramipexole or rotigotine, which are often prescribed for Parkinson's disease. However, these can worsen symptoms over time. Side effects include sleepiness and the potential for compulsive behaviors. Opiate medications like tramadol or oxycodone may also be used, but in low doses due to their side effects, particularly constipation. Finally, anti-anxiety medications like benzodiazepines can be used in severe cases.

It is important to note that all of these treatments need to be taken under the supervision of a healthcare professional and should only be used by consulting a doctor first.

Managing Daytime Fatigue

If you have any of the above-mentioned sleep disorders, daytime fatigue is probably the most difficult symptom for you to manage. Even if you don't have any disorders, the quality of sleep itself declines in PD. If you think about it, Parkinson's is something that makes you slower and stiffer, and it takes a lot of energy to overcome that slowness and stiffness. This can be very fatiguing during the day. First and foremost, fatigue is an enduring tiredness felt both physically and mentally. It is a profound exhaustion that persists even during rest. In contrast, sleepiness is the desire to fall asleep, where closing your eyes may easily lead to drifting off. About 50% of people living with Parkinson's disease experience it, with one-third of them considering it the most debilitating non-motor symptom.

So when does fatigue occur?

It can occur at any stage, early in the diagnosis or after a prolonged period of time. There's no rhyme or reason as to exactly when it can occur. In addition, it can happen regardless of how severe or how mild the movement symptoms are. So, you could hardly have any tremors, maybe just a little bit of slower movements, shuffling gait, things like that, and still have a lot of fatigue.

Conversely, you can have a lot of dystonia, tremors, and a lot of rigidity and not have as much fatigue as some other people. It can also be associated with off times because, with the dopaminergic changes that happen with Parkinson's disease, your energy levels can fluctuate. Sometimes, it's just a matter of addressing the under-treatment of the symptoms that can help with fatigue. On the flip side, sometimes, the medications can be sedating. There can be a side effect of the medication causing sleepiness or sedation during the day.

Another common issue that many individuals with PD face is Depression, a mental health condition that has a significant impact on one's quality of life. It can manifest as feelings of sedation, apathy, and fatigue, which ultimately result in a lack of interest and energy throughout the day.

Finally, Parkinson's symptoms can affect people at night. This is not something that turns off when you go to bed. These symptoms can disrupt your sleep. Not treating your disease appropriately during the nighttime hours can result in disrupted sleep for some people and can certainly make the person's symptoms worse the next day.

Andrew Duker, MD, the director of the Gardner Center for Parkinson's Disease and Movement Disorders, emphasizes the importance of incorporating short naps into your routine. These brief periods of rest, ideally lasting between 30 to 60 minutes, can offer much-needed respite from fatigue. While they may not guarantee complete rejuvenation, even a little bit of rest during the day can help alleviate the feeling of exhaustion.

From a social standpoint, Dr. Duker advises against isolating oneself. The consequences of social isolation are far-reaching and can lead to a negative spiral of increased depression and worsening fatigue. Instead, you should pursue social activities and interactions. This can range from having a friend over for a cup of coffee or tea, enjoying a meal together, or actively participating in Parkinson's support group meetings. Getting involved in social activities not only helps you feel more connected but also keeps you from being too sedentary.

One helpful strategy for managing your day more effectively is to break it down into smaller, manageable chunks. Instead of tackling an entire house project at once, consider breaking it up into smaller tasks. For example, you could vacuum one room at a time or work on different aspects of the project in separate sessions. This approach can be applied not only to household tasks but also to physical or social activities. By planning and engaging in short bouts of activity, you can better pace yourself and prevent burnout.

Remember, it's important to take breaks when working on any physical project — there s no need to push yourself beyond your limits. By incorporating this approach, you can still accomplish a lot while maintaining a balanced and sustainable pace throughout your day.

Another beneficial approach is to plan ahead and schedule tasks in advance. This way, you can ensure that all of your necessary responsibilities are taken care of while still leaving ample time for rest and relaxation. When creating a schedule, be sure to set realistic goals that account for the amount of time and energy you have available each day.

Strategies for Improving Sleep Quality

When it comes to discussing sleep hygiene and identifying the root causes of sleep problems, accurate identification is key to successful treatment. Patients visiting their doctor should be prepared to describe their sleep issues in detail.

1. Is it a problem with falling asleep?
2. Do they struggle to stay asleep with frequent awakenings?
3. Are there any involuntary movements disrupting their sleep?
4. Are there vivid dreams leading to sleep disruptions?

However, it's important to note that most patients have multiple reasons for their disrupted sleep patterns. So, let's delve into some practical pointers that can benefit any sleep-deprived individual.

Start a Healthier Bedtime Routine

Psychologists suggest that having a consistent bedtime and wake time helps establish a regular circadian rhythm. A healthy bedtime routine should involve activities that help to settle the mind and relax the body, such as reading, listening to soothing music, or taking a warm bath. It's also important to avoid stimulants like caffeine and nicotine in the late afternoon or evening because these can make it harder to fall asleep.

Your sleep time has to be regular. You should go to bed at approximately the same time every evening so that you train your brain to be prepared to get relaxed and to get into the mode of falling asleep. Watching TV in the bedroom is not a good idea because that will alert you and distract your brain from preparing for sleep. In addition, it's also important to get up at the same time each day so that you are not throwing off your circadian rhythm.

Reduce Stress and Anxiety

Stress is a common factor that contributes to disruptive sleep patterns. Practicing regular mindfulness exercises such as yoga or meditation can help reduce stress levels and promote better quality sleep. Additionally, minimizing exposure to blue light from electronics at night can help improve sleep quality. Finally, talking to a mental health professional or counselor can be beneficial for managing stress and anxiety in the long term.

Create a Relaxing Environment

Creating a comfortable, dark, quiet environment is essential for better sleep. Investing in blackout curtains or shades, ear plugs, and an eye mask are all great ways to block out distracting light and noise. Ensuring your bedroom is the right temperature and using comfortable bedding can also help create a better sleep environment.

Exercise & Diet

Being physically active helps regulate hormones and improve moods, which in turn can reduce stress levels. Getting regular exercise throughout the day has been linked to better sleep quality and improved sleep duration. Eating a balanced diet with adequate amounts of protein, healthy carbohydrates, and fats can also help reduce stress hormones.

These are some strategies that could help you maintain good, healthy sleep habits. Obviously, sleep problems in Parkinson's can go beyond maintaining good sleep hygiene, and a number of patients will need medications to maintain sleep. However, if you are having difficulty sleeping, it can't hurt to try these techniques first. Remember that everyone is different, and what works for one person may not work for another. Sleep is an essential part of our well-being, and understanding how it works, the ways it can be disrupted, and what strategies you should apply when that happens can prepare you for a healthier lifestyle.

In the next chapter, we will review the communication strategies for PD patients with speech and language difficulties.

Chapter 8: Communication Strategies Guide for Parkinson's Patients and Caregivers

"I remember saying to a lady, it is the uncertainty I can't stand because we don't know how this disease is going to develop, or when it is going to take off. And the person I was speaking to said: 'Anybody who thinks they are living with certainty is kidding themselves. And we all live with uncertainty daily.'" –

Gordon Adair

Imagine having to dredge up all your cognitive ability to first think of what you are trying to say. Then you realize all the words are on the tip of your tongue. But, it takes much longer than what is considered "socially acceptable" to push them out. So, you slowly eke out what you want to say as if you are shouting, only to realize that to other people, it sounds like a feeble whisper. This is the story of many patients with PD. In fact, studies show that those with Parkinson's are more prone to having problems communicating than others. And as if this weren't enough, it can also lead to other complications like depression and social isolation because you cannot easily communicate with people.

More than half of individuals with Parkinson's disease encounter speech difficulties. As a caregiver, you may observe this in the person you're caring for. Alternatively, if you're a loved one, you may notice this as the most challenging aspect for the individual with Parkinson's in your life. These are significant things to talk about because 80% to 90% of Parkinson's patients will have some vocal change. It can be anything from a simple stutter to slurring to volume changes.

And so, understanding these vocal changes is really important and can help identify potential treatments.

Addressing Speech and Voice Changes

An individual with Parkinson's disease may often not be aware that they're experiencing difficulty communicating. Approximately 89 percent of them might not realize that their communication is being affected. This lack of awareness can lead to misperceptions about their own speech, such as believing they are speaking loudly or shouting when, in reality, their speech is quite different from what they intend.

When we communicate, we share meaning through various channels: verbal (talking), non-verbal (facial expressions, body language), and written communication. These different aspects fall under the category of conventional communication, which encompasses general human language. This is why natural gestures and shared intentions play a productive role in communication, as they establish a common ground.

So, what about Parkinson's disease makes communication so challenging?

It all comes down to the combination of cognitive and motor symptoms experienced by patients with Parkinson's. The condition brings about anatomical changes in the dopamine networks, affecting both the frontal area of the brain and the subcortical area. This has an effect on certain aspects of communication, including intentionality. Deciding what to do, when to do it, and then initiating those things. Initiating communication can be impacted. It's difficult for them to start and stop conversations or even hold someone's attention. This is why the primary challenges include

1. Distractibility
2. Inattentiveness
3. Ruminative thoughts

Another challenge is **sequencing thoughts**, which refers to the ability to logically follow and understand conversations in order to respond effectively. All of these cognitive problems are multifaceted but play a significant role in Parkinson's.

In addition, there is **word-finding difficulty**. This is that tip-of-the-tongue phenomenon. You know when you're in the middle of a conversation, and you're talking, and "Oh, that word, it is right there, I can't think of it, but it's on the tip of my tongue." That happens frequently in Parkinson's patients as well. You see this in patients whose primary motor concerns are rigidity and the inability to move.

You can imagine initiating speech movements, among other movements, is a big issue. People often experience a soft, breathy voice and may have difficulty initiating speech movements or controlling the volume. Soft speech, characterized by low volume, is one of the challenges that Parkinson's patients face when trying to communicate effectively. Their speech tends to be too quiet for others to hear clearly, which can lead to misunderstandings and frustrations in conversations.

Another problem associated with communication in Parkinson's disease is changes to the rate of speech. It can be very slow and labored, or it can be very rapid. This happens because the ability to modulate speech movement is affected by slower rates of initiation and the inability to control their volume. Your voice could become soft, you could have a vocal tremor, and many things could happen, including disfluent speech, which can impact your day-to-day life and quality of life.

In addition, patients with Parkinson's may have difficulty finding the right words or understanding what others are saying due to changes in language processing. In some cases, they might not be able to understand complex sentences or conversations if they contain more than one idea or concept. This is because they cannot process multiple ideas simultaneously as easily as they could before the onset of Parkinson's. Additionally, 45% to 50% of patients have articulation deficits. This can include difficulty producing certain sounds or pronouncing words correctly. This can lead to communication errors that could be misinterpreted by family and friends, leading to frustration for the patient.

These changes in speech can contribute to social isolation, depression, and anxiety. Therefore, seeking speech therapy as soon as possible is crucial if you are experiencing any of these issues.

Strategies for Patients to Facilitate Communication

1. Patients with Parkinson's can use these strategies to overcome communication challenges and create a more effective environment for communication:
2. Find alternate ways to express interest: If verbal communication is difficult, use non-verbal cues such as nodding, smiling, or gestures to show that you're engaged and interested. Carrying paper and pen can also be helpful for jotting down thoughts.
3. Speak slowly and use short phrases: Take your time and use simple, concise sentences. Avoid long, complex sentences that might be challenging to articulate. Telegraphic speech, where

you omit unnecessary words, can make communication more efficient.

4. Practice telegraphic speech: Use minimalistic speech that gets the point across without unnecessary words. For example, say "we go" instead of "we need to go." This reduces cognitive demand and can help improve speech clarity.

5. Use visual aids: Visual aids like whiteboards or picture cards can be helpful for communication. If finding the right word is difficult, you can point to a picture or write down keywords to convey your message.

6. Advocate for yourself: Don't hesitate to let others know about your communication challenges. Inform friends, family, and healthcare providers so they can adjust their communication styles and create a supportive environment for you.

7. Take breaks: Conversations can be physically and mentally demanding. It's okay to take breaks during longer conversations to rest and recharge.

By implementing these strategies, patients can enhance their communication skills, reduce frustration, and engage more effectively in conversations.

Alternative Communication Methods

Other than verbal communication, there are alternative methods that might be affected by PD. Non-verbal cues are also incredibly essential for communication. When you are a part of effective communication, you need to be aware of facial expressions and gestures. One challenge comes when individuals have a masked face, where the facial expressions are concealed. When we are unable to discern the thoughts or emotions of others, whether it be a smile or a frown, it can hinder cooperative interaction. The risk of misinterpretation increases without visual cues, making individuals feel unheard or uninterested in the conversation. In my personal experience, I did not realize this fact early on, and it caused many moments of misunderstanding, frustration, and miscommunication.

Additionally, writing is another form of communication that may be affected by PD. Two common symptoms are Micrographia, a condition in which handwriting becomes progressively smaller and more cramped. The second is tremors that cause involuntary shaking, making writing difficult and sometimes illegible. Therefore, it is important to look into alternative communication methods to help patients express themselves effectively without relying solely on writing. For example, voice recognition software can make it easier for patients to dictate their words quickly and accurately.

Augmentative and alternative communication devices like text-to-speech software can also be incredibly useful for those with PD. Such technology can help bridge the gap between nonverbal and verbal expressions, helping patients to communicate more efficiently by providing access to a larger vocabulary of words or even complete sentences. Assistive technologies are also available, such as electronic keyboards and mouse replacements that can reduce the physical stress of typing. These tools can help make communication easier and faster for those with PD.

It is important to note that when choosing the right technology to use, it should take into consideration each patient's individual needs. For example, some patients may find a touchscreen device easier to use than a traditional keyboard or mouse. Additionally, it is important to select technologies that are tailored to the specific needs of those with PD, such as voice recognition software or specialized apps and hardware. By providing access to the right technology, individuals with Parkinson's disease can communicate more effectively and live fuller lives.

Educating Family and Friends about Communication Challenges

Experts say 65% of divorces are due to miscommunication, and a number of pieces they highlight contribute to this miscommunication. These could also overlap with some of those communication deficits that we have in Parkinson's. It is important to understand these communication deficits because if you're a caregiver, your actual ability to be a caregiver directly impacts the Parkinson's patient's outcomes. So, if you're burnt out, you're likely not giving them the care they need, and their outcomes will be worse.

There's also a shift from being super independent to needing more care as the disease progresses. This shift in roles can be challenging. For some people who were once the providers, the ones who took care of everything, now that role has changed. They're not used to asking for things and saying, "Hey, I need this." That shift can cause the caregiver to not specifically know what the patient needs, leading to inefficiencies and confusion in caregiving.

Finally, when it comes to caregivers, the reality is that caregiving is not only emotionally demanding but also comes with an overwhelming financial burden. The responsibility often falls on a close loved one, resulting in a significant role change and added responsibilities. It is crucial to create an open and supportive environment that encourages meaningful communication about these challenges. Caregiving is not just about fulfilling the duties of a caregiver; it is about maintaining a partnership where both parties' physical and emotional needs are acknowledged and addressed. This mutual understanding is equally vital for the well-being of both the caregiver and the patient. Here are some things to remember when trying to foster effective communication.

Communication Strategies for Parkinson's Caregivers:

Actively listen: Give people time to express themselves and avoid rushing them. Just because there are changes, it doesn't mean the person is not there anymore. Just because they can't speak as fast doesn't mean a completely new person is in front of you. So, it's important to put yourself in their shoes.

Take your time with the person speaking. You don't need to hurry. If you're engaged in a casual conversation, give people time.

Speak slowly. This is very important because when we are all trying to communicate and talk fast, we're doing a million things. We're generally increasing our anxiety at a baseline level. This could be anxiety-provoking for a patient with cognitive deficits experiencing vocal production issues. Speaking slowly and clearly can help bridge the gap between patient and provider.

Encourage everyone's involvement in the conversation as well. You can do this if you know the loved one you're talking with has significant vocal deficits or speech problems. Their receptive language is there, meaning their ability to comprehend and understand is intact, but it's the expressive language that's the challenge. So, you can ask closed-ended questions— questions that require a yes or no answer. It's easy to nod your head, shake your head, or say one word.

For caregivers, providers, and families, using **open body language** is important. This can be challenging for patients, but for caregivers, it's essential. When a patient sees you relaxed, engaged, observing them, and actively listening, it can reduce their anxiety and make them feel more comfortable.

Reduce stress: Conversations can be stressful, so create a comfortable and stress-free environment for communication.

As the disease progresses and changes happen, it's really important to keep in constant touch with your loved ones as well. Openly communicate these challenges. Practice communicating with them, saying, "Hey, listen, I'm having a hard time with this. We need to think of strategies so I can let you know in social situations that I'm struggling. Maybe you can intervene or suggest what I can do or how I can express myself better."

Remember, effective communication is a two-way street, and both parties should try to understand and support each other.

Environmental Changes for Effective Communication:

Environmental changes can significantly impact communication, whether in social events or at home. Consider these modifications to create a more conducive environment for effective communication:

1. Reduce background noise: During conversations, turn down the TV and limit any unnecessary background noises that could be distracting. This is particularly important for someone with difficulty projecting their voice.

2. Turn off mobile phones: Mobile phones and social media can be significant distractions. Encourage family members to silence or put away their phones during conversations, especially when someone with Parkinson's is speaking. This shows respect and engagement.

3. Ensure good lighting: Adequate lighting is crucial for understanding facial expressions, lip reading, and body language. Make sure the environment is well-lit so communication cues are easily visible.

4. Use a computer for writing: For individuals with writing difficulties like micrographia or tremors, using a computer can be helpful for written communication. It allows for legible and spell-checked writing, making communication clearer.

These environmental changes can improve communication and make both parties feel more comfortable and engaged in the conversation. It's important to remember that every individual is unique and may require different accommodations. It's always a good idea to ask for feedback from the person with Parkinson's about how best to accommodate their communication needs. Ensuring conversations are enjoyable and effective will help build strong relationships between individuals with Parkinson's disease and those in their lives.

Working with Speech-Language Pathologists

The challenges that both the speaker and the listener can face in communication when someone with Parkinson's disease is involved are numerous. The speaker might feel frustrated due to their perception of repeating themselves and potentially speaking too loudly. At the same time, the listener might struggle to hear and understand due to changes in vocal quality and articulation.

Early intervention through speech therapy is crucial for individuals experiencing difficulty in communication due to Parkinson's disease. Programs like LSVT LOUD (Lee Silverman Voice Treatment LOUD) and SPEAK OUT have been extensively researched and are designed to address these communication challenges. By working with a speech therapist trained in these specialized programs, individuals with Parkinson's can receive targeted intervention to improve their speech, vocal quality, and overall communication abilities.

LSVT LOUD is an incredibly effective speech treatment for individuals diagnosed with Parkinson's disease (PD) and other neurological conditions. It's named after the remarkable Mrs. Lee Silverman (Lee Silverman Voice Treatment), who tenaciously faced PD. Developed by Dr. Lorraine Ramig, this treatment has been rigorously studied for over 25 years with unwavering support from the National Institute for Deafness and Other Communication Disorders within the prestigious National Institutes of Health (NIH), alongside other esteemed funding organizations.

The transformative power of LSVT LOUD lies in training individuals with PD to regain control over their voice, speaking with a more natural and comfortable loudness level in their day-to-day interactions, whether at home, work, or within their community. This treatment is dedicated to assisting individuals in "recalibrating" their perceptions, enabling them to understand how their voice resonates with others and empowering them to confidently use a stronger voice at a normal loudness level.

LSVT LOUD treatment has been helpful for people at all stages of PD, with most research focusing on those at moderate stages of the disease. Additionally, it has shown promise in aiding individuals with atypical parkinsonisms like progressive supranuclear palsy (PSP), and it has also been beneficial for adults with speech issues resulting from stroke or multiple sclerosis, as well as children with cerebral palsy or Down syndrome. Starting it before significant voice, speech, and communication problems arise often leads to the best outcomes, but it's never too late to begin.

SPEAK OUT focuses on the importance of purposeful speech and transforming it from an automatic function to an intentional action. Patients and their speech-language pathologists collaborate on speech, voice, and cognitive exercises to achieve desired results. The ultimate goal of the program is to improve the patient's ability to communicate with others and participate in daily activities.

In the end, LSVT LOUD and SPEAK OUT can provide a range of improvements to PD patients by helping them communicate more effectively and improve their quality of life. With continued practice, patients can experience an improved ability to express themselves, increased motivation, improved self-confidence, and better quality relationships with others.

Be sure you connect with people and take care of other symptoms of PD, too, because outcomes are best for patients who are socially engaged. So, the more socially active you are, the better your outcome. I'll leave you with this quote from George Bernard Shaw:

"The single biggest problem in communication skills is the illusion that it has taken place."

In the next chapter, we'll discuss strategies to help you make financial and legal planning decisions for Parkinson's Disease.

Chapter 9: Financial and Legal Planning Guide for Parkinson's Patients and Caregivers

"I often say now I don't have any choice whether or not I have Parkinson's, but surrounding that non-choice is a million other choices that I can make." –

Michael J. Fox

Living in the present is important. However, it's a fine line between preparing for the future and not over-planning. Careful financial and legal planning can help ensure that you and your family are taken care of in the event of an unexpected situation. Planning for the future in the context of Parkinson's disease is a complex and individualized process. Different factors come into play, making it challenging to predict outcomes with certainty. Nevertheless, it's important to understand the financial implications of Parkinson's so that you can make an informed decision about what will work best for you.

Individuals diagnosed at a younger age need to address issues like maintaining job performance, job security, and possibly early retirement planning. More aggressive treatment might be necessary to ensure productivity is sustained. For those diagnosed in their 50s, 60s, or 70s, the retirement age might be approaching or already upon them. In such cases, it's essential to strike a balance between planning for retirement while staying mindful that the course of the disease can vary widely.

While it's challenging to provide specific advice due to the individual nature of each situation, recognizing the potential timeframes of functional capability can guide decisions. People may have five years of good function or even up to 20, but living in the moment while having some awareness of potential changes is a balancing act that must be tailored to each person's circumstances.

Importance of Financial Planning

A diagnosis of Parkinson's disease can bring financial challenges. It is not unusual for one or both partners to stop working due to the progression of the disease, creating a need to re-evaluate and adjust retirement plans. However, financial planning is nuanced and requires special consideration for Parkinson's patients.

For example, long-term care insurance, which covers home health care and assisted living facilities, may be especially crucial due to the unpredictability of Parkinson's disease progression. Additionally, many people affected by Parkinson's choose to use a financial planner with experience in planning for those with chronic illnesses.

Other things that must be considered include life insurance and investments in retirement accounts, all of which need to be tailored so they can accommodate changes caused by Parkinson's. A financial planner can help you with these tasks, as they have the experience to know when changes need to be made and how best to make them. Here are some of the terms that you should familiarize yourself with when planning:

1. Financial Management: Involves the effective management of finances and resources.
2. Investment Planning: Focuses on developing strategies to invest funds wisely.
3. Insurance and Risk Management: Involves assessing and mitigating potential risks through insurance coverage.
4. Retirement Planning: Involves planning for a financially secure retirement.
5. Tax Planning: Involves minimizing tax liabilities through strategic financial planning.
6. Estate Planning: Deals with managing and distributing one's assets upon their demise.

Out of these, estate planning is more of a blanket term that can involve other aspects of financial planning, such as asset protection, tax minimization strategies, and more. Understanding the different types of estate plans available and how they can benefit you in the long run is important.

Legal Considerations and Advance Directives

When most people hear the words estate planning, they think, 'Oh, I need a will, that's important.' But it's not a significant part of what estate planning really is. It's a much broader process; it has to be more about planning for life than planning for death. I want to be positive and assist you in ensuring your security and safety for the remaining years of your lives. Estate planning is critical in achieving this goal. However, it is important to redefine and broaden our understanding of estate planning beyond the common perception. Ultimately, it is about planning for life and providing peace of mind. That may sound vague, but it really is. Estate planning appropriately done integrates a wide range of different disciplines: your investment planning, insurance planning, practical emergency steps, disability planning, and retirement planning.

If you're living with PD or a loved one has PD, it's almost the same core planning. You don't need an accountant, an attorney, or a will specifically designed for somebody with PD, but every aspect of planning must be modified because it's not tailored to meet the issues of PD generally. It's just specifically for your challenges. So, if you have young onset PD, your situation may differ from somebody 20 or 30 years older.

So, whether you're hiring an expensive estate planning specialist or you're having to use an online website for legal documents, you still want to make sure that the language of those documents reflects the lifestyle and needs of a person with PD. You also want to ensure those documents align with insurance policies, asset management strategies, wills, and other legal documents.

But be mindful that the people you consult with need to understand your challenges and Parkinson's disease before they begin. Don't assume that somebody who has not been touched by PD understands what it does or what it means to you.

When selecting an estate planner, consider their credentials, specialization, and local expertise. Seek recommendations from professionals in related fields and assess their years of experience, reputation, and reviews. Use online resources like the FPA, NAEPC, and Certified Financial Planner Board of Standards to find certified professionals in your area.

When you consult with an attorney, explain what your symptoms are. If you're going to handle this on your own, sit down and maybe even make a list of what your symptoms are and what they might be. Once that is taken care of, start following these steps to make sure that all of your documents are in order.

Step 1: Organize Emergency Financial and Advisor Information

1. Gather all financial and advisor information, including passwords, account numbers, and contact details.
2. Consider using password management apps to securely store and share sensitive information with trusted family members or advisors.
3. Scan and store existing estate planning documents and critical legal papers securely.
4. Compile income and expense information, including budgets and financial statements.
5. Create a comprehensive list of advisor contacts, including lawyers, financial planners, physicians, and others who need to be informed in emergencies.
6. Consider consolidating your investment assets and banking accounts to simplify tracking and management.
7. Set up duplicate monthly statements for key financial accounts to be sent to a trusted family member or CPA.

Having all this information organized and ensuring that someone can access it in an emergency is critical. You need to organize all your investment information because as you age, keeping track of that gets harder and harder. The more simplified and organized things are, the better.

If you consolidate all your assets, you can track them easier, and it's much simpler to manage them. You also want to have someone else who has access to your information in case of an emergency. So, having trusted family members or CPAs set up as a duplicate contact for key financial accounts is a great idea. This way, there is always someone who can access important documents if needed.

Step 2: Create a Budget and Financial Plan

Budgeting is essential. If you run out of money, all the planning in the world is not going to help. Most people hate the process of having to put a budget together. They think it can constrain them. On the contrary, it's empowering. If you have to cut back a little to ensure that you don't run out of money for the last decade of your life, it's well worth it.

1. Develop a detailed budget that accounts for current and projected expenses.
2. Use budgeting tools or software, like QuickBooks or budgeting apps, to track your finances.

3. Review your budget regularly to assess if adjustments are necessary based on changes in your health or financial circumstances.
4. Consider the long-term impact of overspending, even in small amounts, and how it can affect your financial stability over time.
5. Be flexible with your budget, recognizing that some years may require more spending due to health-related expenses.

Remember, financial planning is an ongoing process, and each individual's circumstances are unique. Regularly reviewing and adjusting your financial plan as needed will help you achieve a greater sense of security and peace of mind.

Step 3: Appointing a Power of Attorney

Every adult over the age of 18 should have a power of attorney in case they become incapacitated. It's important to designate someone you trust to handle legal, tax, and financial matters on your behalf. Otherwise, a court may have to intervene, which can be costly and undesirable.

When choosing an agent, consider how much authority you want to give them. If you have full confidence in the agent, that's perfectly fine. The agent will handle financial transactions and legal matters when you cannot. However, if you prefer checks and balances, keeping duplicate statements and involving someone other than the agent whenever possible is a good idea. You can also consider appointing joint agents who must both sign, even though it may be a bit more administratively complex. This can provide an important additional check and balance.

There's another concept that you need to be mindful of called a durable power of attorney; this is the one that remains effective even if you're disabled. A durable power of attorney can be broad or limited in scope, depending on your wishes. You can also grant an agent specific powers, such as the ability to access bank accounts and make decisions about medical care. It's important to recognize that once a document has been signed, it can't be revoked without going through the proper legal channels. That means if you choose to appoint a joint agent, it might be difficult to get rid of that person if it doesn't work out.

One way to mitigate this risk is to include a provision in the document that clarifies that any power granted may be revoked by either party at any time with reasonable notice. This can provide some flexibility and comfort should problems arise. Additionally, you may want to consider including a clause specifying that all decisions must be agreed upon by both agents.

Finally, there are important factors to consider for the power of attorney to be effective. For instance, if you want the best legal power of attorney, but your finances need to be organized as discussed in step one, and your expenses need to be accounted for, how can someone else take over and know what to do?

Let's say you've assigned your oldest daughter as your agent. If she needs to step in and manage your finances, but you have multiple bank accounts, and she has her own family and career, how will she find the time to keep track of everything? Simplify and consolidate.

Did you know 38 percent of women aged 65 and older have their long-term care insurance policies lapse? And the primary reason for policy lapses is failure to pay premiums. These individuals have not organized their finances, signed a power of attorney, or ensured their agent knows what to do. The best way to ensure your loved one can manage your finances is to organize everything.

Step 4: Appoint a Health Proxy

Every adult should have a health proxy to designate someone to make medical decisions. It is important to keep these powers separate from financial power of attorney. Remember to sign the document according to your state's requirements. I recommend having a notary and two witnesses who are not potential beneficiaries of your will, as this could invalidate the document in some states. This ensures the document remains valid even if you move or travel. We will delve further into the nuances of healthcare proxy in the upcoming chapters, including living will, POLST, and other related documents.

Step 5: Protecting Your Child

If you have a child, especially a minor child, you should take steps to protect them. Share child care and medical info in the emergency data we discussed earlier. Also, ensure you've got proper insurance coverage and let others know about it. That way, if you're traveling or get sick and your child needs care, someone's got all the essential details.

Step 6: Finalizing Your Will

Your will has nothing to do with PD. All the other planning involves protecting you and your loved ones in light of PD. But your will is just your will. It's really no different than anyone else's will.

Make sure you have the right people in place to take care of your loved ones if something were to happen. Name trusted family members or friends as executors, guardians for any minor children, and trustees for any trusts you may set up. Have a will that clearly states your wishes regarding what should happen with your property when you pass away. Make sure it is properly signed and witnessed.

It is also important to remember that your will should be reviewed every few years or whenever there is a major life event (like a marriage, divorce, birth of a child, etc.). This way, you can ensure that it still reflects your wishes and considers any changes in your own circumstances or those of your loved ones. With proper planning, you can give your family peace of mind, knowing that all of your wishes will be carried out after you pass away.

In essence, all the steps of estate planning work together to create a comprehensive plan for the future. They ensure that not only your assets are protected but also that those closest to you are taken care of in the event of your death. With thoughtful and proactive estate planning, you can be confident that your wishes will be respected and carried out after you are gone. However, keep in mind that effective planning requires open communication with your chosen representatives. Simply naming them as trustees or agents is not enough. Take the time to have detailed conversations about their roles and responsibilities. Empower them with vital information such as passwords and contact details of professionals involved. By doing so, you can ensure a smooth transition of responsibilities when needed. Proper communication is often overlooked but can make all the difference in successful estate planning.

Understanding Insurance Coverage

As a person with PD, as soon as you hear the word insurance, you probably jump to life insurance. Life insurance is an integral part of estate planning, as it can help to provide for your family in the event of your death. However, there are other types of insurance coverage that should be taken into consideration when considering how to plan one's estate. For example, your property and casualty insurance. Do you have enough coverage if you're struggling with PD and get hurt? What kind of coverage is there? Do you have disability coverage? Do you have long-term care coverage?

If you have **long-term care coverage** and have recently been diagnosed with PD without having made a claim, review your policy. Take a closer look at any disclosure or reporting requirements, and ensure that you have claimed all the benefits you are entitled to but haven't yet utilized.

Disability coverage provides financial protection in the event that you are unable to work due to a disability or illness. If you have disability insurance, it means that you have a policy that can provide you with income replacement if you become disabled and unable to earn an income. It's important to review your policy and understand the claims process to ensure that you can effectively utilize this powerful tool. Additionally, even if you don't qualify for new insurance, it's worth checking if you have existing coverage that can offer you the protection you need.

Liability coverage is crucial, regardless of whether your PD affects your driving ability. Imagine being in an accident and the other party's lawyer discovering you have PD; they may falsely argue it caused the accident. To protect yourself, ensure you have substantial liability coverage. Whether you own a house or drive a car, it's wise to have excess liability insurance since standard policies often have limited coverage. Considering PD, it becomes even more vital. Adding a few million dollars of coverage to your personal excess liability policy is usually affordable.

The key point is to look at all of your insurance coverage, not only from the perspective of PD but from the broad perspective of whether you have everything you need and if you're taking full advantage of what you can.

Long-Term Care Options For Parkisnon's

Long-term care is not easy. And it's definitely not inexpensive. However, there are options available that can help provide assistance and support to individuals living with Parkinson's.

One option is **long-term care insurance**, which can help with ongoing medical care, home health aides, and other services for people with Parkinson's. The premiums for this insurance may be high, but it's usually worth the cost. These policies are typically activated when there is a significant need for care. Some long-term care insurance policies cover in-home care, while others only cover skilled nursing facilities. In progressive diseases like PD, the services covered can be used up quickly, so it's important to carefully evaluate the benefits and limits.

Medicaid is a government service that offers healthcare coverage to low-income individuals, those with disabilities, and recipients of federally assisted income maintenance payments like Supplemental Security Income. It includes coverage for nursing home care, waivers for home-based care, and support for personal care attendants or paid caregivers.

Veterans Affairs benefits are for current and retired military personnel. The VA provides comprehensive services, ensuring that veterans receive the support they deserve, whether the physical or mental disability is directly connected to their time in service or not. From healthcare and rehabilitation programs to education and housing assistance, the VA is committed to improving the lives of our honored veterans.

The **Melvin Weinstein Parkinson's Foundation** is an alternative resource that offers financial aid to eligible individuals with PD. Their funds can provide assistance for home health care and essential medical equipment like walkers, wheelchairs, and canes.

Finally, the **Parkinson's Wellness Fund** is dedicated to supporting individuals living with PD and their caregivers by providing essential grants for a wide range of healthcare services. These grants are conveniently distributed as vouchers, which can be redeemed for services through an extensive network of highly qualified and compassionate professionals.

While these long-term benefits are an important lifeline for those living with PD, there are disability benefits available to compensate those who are no longer able to work.

Navigating Disability Benefits and Social Security

Disability benefits may be available to you if you are physically unable to work due to an injury or illness. These benefits can help support you financially while you take time off to recover, receive treatments, and adjust your life accordingly.

Social Security is another excellent resource that can provide financial assistance for people with disabilities. The two most common types of Social Security benefits are Retirement and Disability Insurance. Each provides its own set of qualifications as to who can receive payments, so it is important to understand the requirements of each before applying.

Additionally, you may be able to find other programs and services that could help you while navigating your disability. For example, Medicaid provides comprehensive health coverage for individuals with limited income and resources; Medicare offers health insurance to individuals over 65 and those with specific disabilities; and Vocational Rehabilitation can provide job training and assistance for those recovering from a disability.

Social Security Disability Insurance (SSDI) is a government benefit program that provides monthly payments to disabled workers who meet specific criteria. It's administered by the Social Security Administration (SSA) and primarily covers total disability, excluding partial or short-term disability. So, if you're wondering about the eligibility for SSDI, keep in mind that it's designed to support those who cannot work due to their disability. In order to qualify for Social Security disability benefits as a person with PD, you need to meet specific criteria outlined in the SSA's medical listing 11.06 for Parkinsonian Syndrome. These criteria include:

1. Demonstrating significant slowness of movement (bradykinesia), rigidity, or tremors in at least two extremities
2. Experiencing prolonged difficulty in movement or walking at an abnormal rate.

Once you have reflected on your symptoms, you need to fill out a form. When filling out your application, you'll need to describe your symptoms and impairments, list your treatment providers, and include any extra information related to your disability. It's a good idea to prepare and organize the necessary information in advance. The SSA provides an Adult Disability Starter Kit to assist you in getting organized for your application.

It's a good idea to chat with your doctors about your Parkinson's disease symptoms and how they affect your ability to work. While your doctors' opinions alone may not be sufficient to win your claim, they are valuable evidence that can support your case. Your doctors will need to provide certification of your disability to the SSA by documenting your symptoms in their examination reports, tests, and claim forms.

You will also need to gather information from other specialists (such as a physical therapist or psychiatrist) and submit any records of hospitalizations, surgeries, treatments, or medications you have received for your disability. Additionally, if you receive treatment from a mental health professional, such as a psychologist or social worker, make sure to include the details in your application form. If applicable, you may also need to submit education records indicating how your disability has affected your ability to function in the classroom. If you can provide sufficient evidence of your condition and its impact on your daily life, the SSA may approve your claim.

Finally, a good idea is to document any efforts you have made to accommodate or manage your disability. For example, if you have enrolled in a vocational program or joined a support organization, provide evidence of your commitment. Doing so may help demonstrate to the SSA that you are taking responsibility for managing your disability and attempting to lead an independent life.

By now, you should be aware of how important financial planning is, what the legal implications of your disability are, and how you can use insurance coverage to your advantage. With the proper amount of preparation and research, you can ensure that you are well-informed and financially secure when it comes to managing a disability. In the next chapter, we will go over some tips on how you can travel safely with PD and manage the unique challenges that come along with it.

Chapter 10: Travel and Leisure Guide for Parkinson's Patients and Caregivers

"I don't dwell on the past or worry about the future. I try to live for today, and Parkinson's hasn't changed that." –

Actor Valerie Perrine

The best thing a person who has been brought down one too many times by Parkinson's can do is take some time off, relax, and enjoy life. Obviously, this is not some advice to bury your head in the sand and ignore the disease, far from it. In this chapter, we'll look at some of the best ways to enjoy yourself and stay positive while managing a chronic health condition.

Traveling can be tricky for even the most experienced traveler, let alone for someone with a chronic condition. It can be stressful and uncomfortable. And if you are traveling somewhere you haven't been before, you may be worried about the unknown. But just because it might be difficult does not mean we shouldn't be doing it. In fact, some studies suggest that traveling can help reduce stress and depression, both of which are common issues associated with Parkinson's. Then again, it can also increase stress and exacerbate symptoms. Then what should we do?

The key is to plan ahead and make sure you are prepared. Let's look at some of the more common problems that you can face when traveling with PD and how you can deal with them.

Tips for Safe and Comfortable Travel

The best way to make sure that you are not caught unawares is to plan ahead and make sure that you are prepared for anything. The most important arsenal of a PD patient is their medications.

Medication & Prescription

Before starting your plan for the trip, have a conversation with your doctor. They should be able to provide you with all the medications and supplies that you will need. They understand the need for you to be able to handle your symptoms and may be able to provide you with a medical kit or other resources that will help. It's also important for you to bring enough medication for the duration of the trip, as well as any additional medications that may be needed in an emergency. Make sure you are familiar with how your medication works and know what to do if something goes wrong. You should keep medications and medical supplies in their original containers, as this will make it much easier for them to be recognized at customs when crossing borders. Be sure to bring a copy of your prescription and the contact information for your doctor with you on the trip.

When you find yourself in a different time zone, it's important to resist the urge to alter your medication timing. Instead, stick to your regular dosing schedule even while traveling, particularly during long train or airline journeys. One effective strategy is to set an alarm to help you remember when it's time to take your dose. This way, you can ensure that you maintain the consistency necessary for optimal medication effectiveness regardless of your location.

It is also recommended to store at least one day's dosage of medication in a fanny pack, pocket, or purse for easy accessibility and convenience. This ensures that you have your medication on hand whenever you need it, giving you peace of mind and reducing the risk of missing a dose while you are out and about.

Destination Selection

Once you have the green light from your healthcare provider, you can start planning your trip. The first questions you should ask yourself are: who is going with you, and where are you going?

Going on a trip with someone you know is always preferred, as it is safer and you have someone to look after you in an emergency. They should know all of your medical conditions and any allergies you may have.

When selecting travel destinations, it is important to prioritize accessibility and convenience. Look for cities that boast well-developed infrastructure, reliable public transportation options, and meticulously maintained sidewalks and pathways. Taking into consideration the prevailing climate is also crucial, as extreme temperatures or high humidity levels can significantly impact your comfort and mobility during your trip.

Furthermore, it is advisable to choose a destination that aligns with your specific needs and requirements. For instance, if you heavily rely on public transportation or require accommodations such as ramps for easy access, it is imperative to consider these factors as you make your decision. Conduct thorough research to ensure that the chosen destination not only meets your mobility prerequisites but also provides a fulfilling and enjoyable experience.

When you are thoroughly researching your destination, it is crucial to proactively prepare for any potential emergencies that may arise. One approach is to conduct detailed research on the local hospitals and medical facilities available at your intended destination. Having this valuable information at hand will empower you to promptly seek medical assistance should the need arise.

Moreover, it is highly recommended to carry a comprehensive list of emergency contacts. This list should include not only your primary care physician's contact details but also any pertinent local contacts you may have access to. In the event of an emergency, having these essential contact numbers readily available can expedite the process of obtaining the necessary medical support, ensuring your well-being and peace of mind throughout your trip.

Also, don't forget to get travel insurance that includes medical emergencies, trip cancellations, and travel disruptions. Make sure the policy covers pre-existing medical conditions.

Accommodation & Accessible Destinations

After deciding on the area you want to visit, it is important to research the lodging options available in the vicinity. Depending on your budget and personal preferences, it is highly recommended to prioritize hotels or accommodations that are wheelchair-friendly. Look for establishments that provide amenities such as ramps, elevators, and accessible rooms to ensure a comfortable and convenient stay that caters to your specific accessibility needs.

When inquiring about bathroom facilities, it is important to specifically mention the need for essential safety features such as grab bars, which provide support and stability. This way, you will know which assistive devices and equipment are available for you to use. Additionally, ask about the availability of accessible parking and ask to be directed to a designated area that is close to your room. You may also want to consider choosing locations that are conveniently located near medical facilities, just in case of any unforeseen emergencies that may arise.

Additionally, research local attractions and activities to ensure they meet your comfort and mobility requirements. When selecting restaurants and venues, prioritize wheelchair accessibility and suitable seating arrangements for those with mobility challenges. Call these establishments and nearby destinations while making accommodation arrangements to confirm their accessibility.

Once you have decided on your destination, research public and private transportation options available for disabled travelers. Whether you choose to rent a car, book an accessible shuttle service, or rely on public transit like buses and trains, make sure that the transport you choose has accommodations suitable for your specific disability needs. Look into wheelchair-friendly taxi services as well, which can be incredibly helpful in easily getting around.

Lastly, don't forget to check reviews online from other guests who have previously stayed at the establishment to get an idea of their experience with accessibility features and overall satisfaction.

Transportation:

Once you've determined your destination, it's time to choose the best transportation option to suit your needs. If you're traveling by air, it's important to ensure you have a seat with ample legroom. Additionally, it's advisable to get up and walk around periodically during the flight to prevent the formation of blood clots in your legs, which can be a serious concern. In case you need assistance while flying, whether it's in the restroom or elsewhere, don't hesitate to ask for help from fellow passengers or airline staff.

When booking your flights, it's a good idea to request assistance in advance for boarding, deplaning, and navigating the airport. You might also consider arranging for special assistance at the airport, such as wheelchair service or an electric cart for help with your luggage. For example, when my wife and I went to Brazil, the airline staff was incredibly helpful during the long flight, deplaning, customs, and getting to our connecting flight. Keep in mind that some airlines may require a physician's certificate of need, so be sure to contact the airline beforehand to confirm any requirements or arrangements.

Ground travel is a great choice for those who enjoy scenic views, meeting new people, and extra legroom. You'll have full access to the radio, so you can create your playlist or catch up on news and entertainment. Adjusting the seats and controlling the interior temperature ensures optimal comfort throughout the journey. Roll down the windows for a sense of freedom and fresh air. Traveling with a chosen companion, like a care partner, family member, or friend, allows for quality time and shared experiences.

Compared to other modes of transportation, traveling by car usually involves fewer or no security protocols, making it more convenient and less time-consuming. Plus, it's easy to stop, stretch your legs, and explore roadside attractions. If you are taking a road trip, then make sure that you take frequent breaks on your way. It's a good idea not to be seated in one place for long durations, and frequent stops allow you the opportunity to walk around and stretch your legs. This can also help you to stay energetic throughout the journey.

Trains are also a great option for individuals with Parkinson's to explore new destinations and connect with others. They offer ample opportunities for movement, helping to maintain mobility. Additionally, the relaxed and comfortable environment can be beneficial for those with Parkinson's who may feel anxious or overwhelmed in unfamiliar settings.

Buses stop approximately every 3 hours for new passengers boarding and current passengers alighting. Most buses have wheelchair lifts and personnel to assist with luggage. Additionally, buses offer ample legroom, often have a restroom onboard, and allow you to request to sit beside your companion or travel partner.

Cruises, however, can be anxiety-inducing for those with Parkinson's. Firstly, the security screening before boarding the ship can be as thorough as air travel, especially since most cruises venture into international waters. Make sure to have your documents in order and keep your medications in their proper containers. Another challenge is the motion of the boat at sea. Always have a care partner or use assistance provided by the cruise to help you maintain stability when leaving your cabin. Most cruises should provide wheelchair accessibility, but it's a good idea to confirm this in advance. You may need special permits or documentation for motorized assistive devices. Additionally, consider booking an "accessible" or "modified" stateroom before making your reservation.

Packing Per Needs

So, you have decided on a course and made all the necessary bookings. What's left to do? Pack for your trip, of course! Pack according to your individual needs, and don't forget any prescriptions. If you are at that stage where you are more reliant on assistive devices such as walkers or wheelchairs, then remember to have the necessary equipment on hand and readily available. And when taking an assistive device, try to envision if it will be usable where you're going. For example, if you decide to take your electric toothbrush with you, make sure that it is compatible with the electric socket of the country where you are going.

It is important to be prepared when you are out and about by having a backup supply of batteries, spare parts, and tools in case something goes wrong. If you have a DBS device, remember to bring the Medtronic device wallet card or the equivalent from your device manufacturer, as you may be asked for it. When dealing with security personnel, it is best to simply mention that you have a medical device or even specifically mention that you have a pacemaker, which they commonly encounter. Keep in mind that you should not go through the old-style security check machines or allow them to use wands for checking. You should be prepared for a pat down if necessary. If you don't have a handicap placard, get one.

When packing, utilize a label maker to clearly mark your name and cell number on loose items like canes. Additionally, remember to bring weather-appropriate clothing for your destinations. Lastly, keep your device wallet card and a copy of your patient profiles, medication list, and travel letter with you at all times.

Here are some extra tips to optimize your travel experience.

1. While exploring new places, consider exploring local Parkinson's offerings, too.
2. If possible, travel with companions who understand you so well that they know when to provide help and when to give you space. They understand when you need rest and when you're ready to go. Most importantly, they can gracefully handle the unpredictability of Parkinson's without letting it hinder your fabulous trip.
3. Maintain a sense of humor. Travel can be challenging, even under the best circumstances. When something goes wrong (and it usually does), how you handle it will significantly impact your physical and emotional well-being. Eventually, you'll get to your destination, so in the meantime, have a good laugh about it.

4. Don't hesitate to let your travel companion know when you're too tired for certain activities and just need some rest. If you can, treat yourself to luxuries and conveniences while traveling. They're designed to make your life easier, and when you're on the road, you deserve that comfort.

Enjoying Leisure Activities with Parkinson's

While the purpose of travel can vary from person to person, leisure activities play a big part for many. And amidst planning the trip, going on the trip, and remembering to take medication correctly, we often forget to have fun and make memories together. It's important to choose activities that fit with your energy level and physical abilities. Here are a few ideas:

1. Swimming is a fantastic form of aerobic exercise that not only gets your heart pumping but also offers a low-impact workout. Unlike walking or running, swimming puts minimal strain on the body, making it an excellent option for people on a vacation with Parkinson's.
2. The beach is a great place to relax and get away from it all. Whether you're looking for a peaceful morning stroll on the shore or an afternoon of kayaking, there are plenty of activities to enjoy while taking in the breathtaking scenery around you.
3. If you like the outdoors, take some time to explore nature trails or parks that are wheelchair-accessible. Wildlife watching and birding offer an excellent way to connect with nature and observe animals in their natural habitat.
4. For a more leisurely activity, try fishing or boating. The calming motion of the boats can help to reduce stress, and the gentle rocking of the waves can be very soothing. Plus, you'll make some great memories while spending time in nature.
5. Finally, for a truly spectacular experience, take a hot air balloon ride and observe the world from a bird's eye view.

Some days, you may not have the energy for physical activity. Watching a movie together is a great way to share an experience without putting any physical strain. Likewise, board games are an excellent way to engage with your family and friends. Whether it's a classic like Monopoly or a modern game like Catan, board games can be fun for everyone. Finally, no trip would be complete without exploring the local culture through food. Taste the unique flavors of the region by trying out new restaurants or visiting the local market for fresh produce.

Lastly, while many things may be beyond your control when traveling, you can control your own experience. Don't let Parkinson's stop you from exploring the world. As Jill Ater wisely said,

"Most people in the world are incredibly understanding and patient. If you love to travel, then it's a part of living fully with Parkinson's."

Remember, the reason why you took the trip is to create memories. Embrace the moments, and don't be afraid to kick back and relax. You planned everything from your itinerary to your destination and accommodations. Make sure you take full advantage of everything the trip has to offer. In the end, you will have these memories to cherish no matter how your Parkinson's journey progresses. Enjoy the journey!

Chapter 11: Palliative Care and End-of-Life Guide for Parkinson's Patients and Caregivers

"My dad had Parkinson's and arthritis, which meant a lot of stiffness. It was extremely difficult to get anyone to treat his pain. At that point, I didn't know palliative care even existed, so I did not know to ask about it — and no one suggested it. In hindsight, if we had access to palliative care, we could have managed his pain better, and his overall quality of life."

- Kelly Weinschreider, person with Parkinson's and care partner

A hundred percent of us die, and yet, despite that, we don't tend to acknowledge that our lives are finite. We often plan for events like birthdays, weddings, anniversaries, and graduations, but we frequently avoid planning for the possibility of living with serious illness, frailty, and incapacity. Most of us don't plan well for our end of life—where we want to be, who we want to have with us, and how we want our death to be acknowledged.

Do we want a funeral?

What do we want to be said?

When we engage in these discussions, I think people tend to pull back, questioning why we're even bringing it up. The reason is that it's important, and the gift we give to those we love is planning for something that might not be comfortable or welcome. Each of us must confront the reality of our mortality, and it makes sense to acknowledge and address our feelings and concerns about what we would want to happen in the event of our passing. Having open conversations about our fears, worries, and desires related to the end of life is a significant step toward ensuring that our wishes are respected and honored. This is a part of the broader concept of advance care planning, which involves making decisions about medical treatments, interventions, and other preferences in the event that we are unable to communicate our choices ourselves.

So, how do you know what you need and when? When should you start thinking about it? When should you access different services, and what are they?

I want you to consider for a moment where you want to be. Who do you want to be with during such times? What's important to you in that vulnerable period? How do you want to manage it? Ideally, how do you want to direct it? Because when we're seriously ill, the only way we can control it is if we do it now before we reach a point where we're so debilitated that we can't. Drawing from personal experience, I can say that one of the most helpful things we can do is plan, discuss, and be open. This is a tough subject to think about and even tougher to talk about, but it is necessary. Circumstances can change quickly, and having a game plan gives you a little control while everything else spins into chaos around you.

Hospice Care and Support Services

The current model of healthcare has a "warrior" model, where providers see diseases as adversaries to conquer, and the focus is primarily on finding cures. We tend to categorize people into various diagnoses and, unfortunately, assign different doctors to each diagnosis. In this process, the person suffering can often get lost amidst the fight against illness. This perspective uses harsh terms like "*fighting illness*," and there's collateral damage associated with this approach. Unfortunately, by viewing individuals through the lens of disease, their personal story, their values, what matters to them, and their connections with loved ones does not get integrated into care. Because if we're constantly fighting, we and our families often become collateral damage.

In the post-World War II era, Dr. Cicely Saunders recognized an opportunity to develop a care model that contrasted with the growing disease-driven approach. She began her career as a nurse, became a social worker after a back injury, and later pursued medicine. Had she pursued spiritual care certification, she could have constituted an entire interdisciplinary team herself.

It's important to note that Saunders didn't invent hospice care, but she is the creator of the modern hospice movement. This movement not only emphasized the art of caring for those at the end of life but also supported the scientific study of providing care for individuals with advanced diseases and those nearing death. She introduced scientific rigor to the care of the dying, a significant development that continues to shape how we approach end-of-life care today.

The primary goals of hospice care are to **alleviate suffering** and **enhance the quality of life** during a finite period of time. Typically, individuals in hospice care are no longer pursuing disease-directed treatments, as the potential benefits of those treatments are outweighed by the burdens they bring. Hospice care shifts the focus to the whole person— addressing their physical, mental, and spiritual needs—as well as the needs of their family and caregivers. It's also about **preparing for death**.

Hospice care is introduced when the prognosis suggests that a patient is more likely to pass away within the coming months. During this critical time, the focus shifts towards managing symptoms and alleviating discomfort rather than treating the underlying illness, which could potentially exacerbate the symptoms. Functional changes, weight loss, difficulties with swallowing, and cognitive changes such as memory recall and clear thinking are critical triggers for initiating hospice care. As the family's ability to care for their loved one becomes increasingly strained, anxieties and fears about navigating this challenging period arise. It is important to recognize these signals and involve professionals who can provide the necessary assistance, offering both support and empathy.

When Cicely Saunders introduced the hospice care model, she initially started it as an inpatient service. Hospices, especially Saint Christopher's Hospice in London, UK, provided specialized care for individuals at the end of life. Saunders' clinical work paved the way for research and education in the science of caring for the dying. This model gained significant traction during the 1950s and 1960s in London and England.

Florence Wald, the Dean of Nursing at Yale University in Connecticut, caught wind of this model and collaborated with Saunders. In 1975, they launched a demonstration project to bring hospice care to the United States. Interestingly, this model quickly shifted towards a home care approach instead of an institution-based one. It evolved into a visiting nurse-driven model, offering care within patients' homes. This demonstration project was groundbreaking, leading to the creation of a group of individuals who championed the cause. In 1982, it even became a demonstration project at the level of Medicare, and by 1986, it was signed into law, officially establishing the hospice care model in the United States.

Personally, in the last two months of my wife's life, We brought in a hospice team. She was frail, suffering from dementia, and needed more help than I could provide alone. I initially had rejected hospice as an option because I did not understand that it was not about giving up. It was about providing the best care possible. The hospice team was wonderful, and I am so glad we decided to call them in.

Medicare Hospice Benefit

When one becomes part of a Medicare program, especially in the context of hospice care, there are mixed blessings. Hospice is a philosophy of care, whereas Medicare is a federally regulated insurance program. When these two meet, there can be limitations in expressing the full philosophy of care due to regulations and funding requirements.

Medicare hospice regulations fall under the Conditions of Participation, which are laws outlined in the Code of Federal Regulations. These laws are decided upon by Congress. According to the benefit, a person is eligible for **two 90-day periods** initially and unlimited 60-day periods thereafter, as long as they remain eligible. Many commercial insurance programs follow the Medicare hospice benefit and have adopted similar structures. Medicaid also follows a similar approach, though there might be variations in coverage compared to commercial insurance.

To be eligible for hospice care, a person must be certified as terminally ill, meaning they have a prognosis of less than six months. Once they're certified, they can choose to use their Medicare hospice benefit to get care. The hospice program also needs to be Medicare-certified. The care covered by the Medicare hospice benefit is comprehensive and robust, making it one of the significant benefits that Medicare offers.

Understanding Palliative Care for Parkinson's Patients

Here is a very significant question: Why do we often wait until people are at the end of their lives to discuss the quality of life, its meaning, and how to best support it with the input of the medical team? This dilemma is common, and many others have raised the same question.

One model that emerged to address this issue was proposed by Dr. Balfour Mount, a urologic surgeon at McGill University in Montreal. He is the physician who coined the term "palliative" to describe this care model. Mount originally trained as an oncologic surgeon at Memorial Sloan Kettering and then traveled to the UK to work with Dame Cicely Saunders to learn about the hospice model. When he brought this knowledge back to

Montreal, he faced the challenge of introducing this concept in a French-speaking environment where the term "hospice" could be misleading due to its association with halfway houses. As a result, he coined the term "palliative care." Through his work and collaboration with Saunders, the field of palliative medicine began to take shape and expand in the UK and Canada. By 1990, this approach began to gain more formal recognition and acceptance in the United States as well.

The delay in discussing the quality of life, meaning, and comprehensive support in healthcare likely stems from historical medical paradigms and a focus on disease treatment. However, the efforts of individuals like Dr. Balfour Mount and the growth of the palliative care movement have aimed to shift this paradigm and emphasize holistic care throughout a person's medical journey, not just at the end of life. The application of whole-person care is not only needed but also essential and life-giving. Palliative care is a specialized holistic model of healthcare designed for individuals with serious illnesses. Importantly, these individuals do not necessarily need to be at the end of life, but they are, by definition, seriously ill. Serious illness in this context refers to conditions that not only increase the risk of mortality but also lead to functional impairments and additional stress on their caregiving system.

Palliative care operates as interdisciplinary and team-based care. It involves clinicians who are experts in managing symptoms, taking a comprehensive view of the person and their family, providing emotional, psychological, and spiritual support as necessary, and helping navigate the complex healthcare system. It aids in making difficult medical decisions, weighing the burden and benefit of various interventions. It's integrated from the very moment of a serious diagnosis and provides support throughout the entire trajectory of the disease. This approach shifts the care model from being solely **disease-directed** to being **person-directed**, encompassing the person's needs and values along with those of their family.

However, palliative medicine and supportive care are distinct from hospice care. While hospice care is a form of palliative care, it's supported by a specific insurance benefit that patients at the end of life can elect to use. In order to access hospice care, individuals must be certified as terminally ill, and it typically involves a team-based approach. Generally, hospice patients are no longer receiving disease-directed treatments as they are no longer considered beneficial for their condition.

To give you a mental picture, think of it like a Venn diagram: all hospice care falls under palliative care, but not all palliative care is hospice care. When someone gets a serious illness diagnosis, palliative care kicks in, providing team-based support. The level of support can change based on their and their family's needs throughout their illness, which could last for months or even years. Moving to hospice care is a gradual process, ensuring individuals and their families have the necessary support towards the end of life. Plus, hospice care doesn't just end after death. It continues to offer bereavement and grief support to those who survive the loss. This support is crucial because it recognizes the ongoing impact of loss on loved ones.

Making Decisions about End-of-Life Care

A vivid analogy for modern healthcare versus interdisciplinary and palliative care is the difference between swimming in lanes and synchronized swimming. In modern healthcare, each discipline sticks to its own "lane," focusing on its tasks and responsibilities. In contrast, palliative and hospice care are more like synchronized swimming, where the person and their family are at the center, and there's coordination, collaboration, and communication happening all around them. It's a more integrative and holistic approach.

To set the stage for this approach, it's essential to understand that it's part of a continuum, and there are crucial milestones to engage with when living with a severe illness. **Planning** is a significant aspect of this continuum, and a crucial element of planning is establishing advanced directives. Despite the importance of this work, more than 80% of people recognize its significance, but fewer than 25% actually document or have conversations about their wishes for care in advanced illness scenarios. This highlights the need for more proactive discussions and planning to ensure that loved ones know what to do in the context of far-advanced illness.

This is where the notion of advance directives comes in. An advance directive is a legal document that allows an individual to state in writing their wishes for care and treatment in the event of incapacity, such as when they can no longer make decisions on their own. This document usually includes instructions for care if the person becomes terminally ill or enters into a persistent vegetative state from which they cannot recover.

There are various types of advanced directives available, including living wills and healthcare power of attorney documents. However, it can be hard to determine which is most appropriate to support the continuum of care. Here's a breakdown of some common options:

Living Will: A living will is a traditional advanced directive that outlines your healthcare preferences, especially regarding treatments you would want or not want in the event of serious illness or incapacity. It often comes into play when someone is terminally ill. However, a living will can be somewhat limiting because it provides guidance but doesn't offer actionable instructions.

Five Wishes: Five Wishes is an advanced directive document created by Jim Tui, who was Mother Teresa's lawyer. This document goes beyond simply stating what treatments you don't want and delves into the things that would bring you comfort and joy in those circumstances. It provides space for detailing preferences related to specific comforts, pleasures, and even small joys that can enhance your quality of life. It allows you to express not only what medical treatments you would or would not want but also your personal preferences and desires for comfort and joy. For instance, you can specify preferences about music, sensory experiences, foods you enjoy, and other factors that contribute to your well-being and happiness.

By incorporating both medical preferences and personal comforts, it creates a more nuanced understanding of your wishes. This can be particularly valuable for your loved ones and caregivers, as it helps them support not just your medical needs but also your emotional and psychological well-being during times of serious illness.

Healthcare Power of Attorney: A healthcare power of attorney, also known as a surrogate decision maker, is a person you designate to make medical decisions on your behalf if you're unable to do so yourself. This individual becomes your voice and advocate, ensuring that your preferences and wishes are followed, especially during times of severe illness or incapacity. This is why it's essential to carefully consider who you designate as your healthcare power of attorney.

1. Designating the Right Person: Your healthcare power of attorney should be someone who truly understands your values and wishes regarding medical care. This person should be at least 18 years old and ideally be someone who can advocate for you according to your preferences, even if those preferences differ from their own.

2. Creating the Document: The process of creating a healthcare power of attorney document is straightforward. You don't need a lawyer or notary to complete it. The document should be created in front of a witness (not the designated person) and signed. It outlines the authority the designated person has to make medical decisions on your behalf.

3. Content of the Document: The healthcare power of attorney document authorizes your chosen representative to interact with healthcare professionals, provide consent for medical tests and treatments, and advocate for your preferences in various medical and end-of-life situations. It's a comprehensive document that gives your chosen person the legal authority to make decisions based on your wishes.

4. Distribution of Copies: It's crucial to share copies of the healthcare power of attorney document with your healthcare providers, doctors, and any relevant individuals. This ensures that your preferences are known and respected in various medical contexts.

5. Availability and Changes: It's advised not to keep the document in a safe deposit box where it might be inaccessible during a medical emergency. You should have copies readily available and let key individuals know where to find them. Remember that you can change your healthcare power of attorney designation at any time by creating a new document. Overall, the healthcare power of attorney empowers a trusted person to serve as your representative, making critical medical decisions in alignment with your wishes when you're unable to do so yourself. This document provides peace of mind and helps ensure your healthcare journey is guided by your values and preferences.

Without a designated health care power of attorney, the state's default order of **surrogacy** will come into play. This order establishes who will be your decision-maker based on a predefined hierarchy, such as spouse, guardian, adult children, and so on. However, this process can become complicated, especially if there are multiple adult children or family members who may have differing opinions. That is why even if your adult children know you well, they may not have the legal authority to make decisions on your behalf without the proper documentation. Designating a healthcare power of attorney ensures that the person you trust most is legally empowered to advocate for your preferences, communicate with medical professionals, and make decisions aligned with your wishes. Creating a healthcare power of attorney simplifies the process and helps prevent potential conflicts or confusion among family members. It's a proactive step that gives you control over who will speak for you when you can't speak for yourself and ensures that your values and choices are honored.

Next, the **Physician Orders for Life-Sustaining Treatment (POLST)** form is a crucial and actionable document that provides medical orders for emergency medical personnel to follow regarding your preferences for life-sustaining treatments. Unlike other advance care planning documents like living wills, this form is specifically designed to provide actionable guidance in emergency situations, especially when paramedics and other emergency medical personnel need to make quick decisions.

Individuals with serious illnesses need to understand that while advance directives like living wills express preferences, the POLST form translates those preferences into **actionable medical orders** that can be honored in real-time emergency situations. The form allows you to specify the level of medical intervention you desire in various situations, ranging from full aggressive treatment to comfort-focused care. It's an essential tool for ensuring that your wishes are respected even when you can't communicate them directly to medical professionals. By completing a POLST form, you're providing clear and legally binding instructions that can guide paramedics and emergency medical personnel in delivering care that aligns with your values and preferences. This helps prevent unwanted interventions or treatments that might be contrary to your wishes.

Now, signing a couple of documents isn't enough. You must engage in ongoing conversations with your loved ones and healthcare providers about your wishes, values, and goals for care. Going a step further, it is also essential to periodically review and update your advanced care planning documents to ensure that they accurately reflect your current preferences and situation. Life is ever-changing, and your healthcare preferences may evolve over time.

By taking the time to review and update your documents, you can have peace of mind knowing that your wishes will be respected and upheld in the unfortunate event that you are unable to communicate them yourself. Stay proactive and keep your advanced care planning up-to-date to ensure your voice is heard and your values are honored.

Benefits of Advanced Care Planning

Advanced care planning is a critical step in ensuring that individuals receive the care they truly want and need, particularly when facing serious illness or the end of life. It goes beyond just medical treatments and interventions—it's about defining your values and goals for care. Here are some key benefits and steps associated with advanced care planning:

Improving Quality of Care:

One of the key benefits of advanced care planning is that it ensures the care provided is in line with the patient's unique preferences and values. This leads to a significant enhancement in the quality of care delivered, resulting in a more personalized and satisfactory experience for the patient. It empowers individuals to **actively participate** in decisions about their healthcare journey, fostering a sense of control and emotional well-being.

Reducing Medical Errors:

Another benefit of advanced care planning is that because it allows individuals to document their preferences and directives, it prevents unwanted or inappropriate medical interventions. By doing so, the risk of errors or complications arising from such interventions is significantly reduced.

Providing Standardization:

Advance directives, such as healthcare power of attorney, living wills, and POLST forms, give straightforward and standardized instructions to healthcare professionals in various settings and situations. This enables healthcare providers to better focus on the patient's individual needs rather than have to guess at what the patient would want.

Maintaining Control:

PD is a disease that can make you feel like you're losing control over your body and life. Writing down your wishes for medical care ahead of time can give you a sense of empowerment and control, knowing that your wishes will be respected if you are no longer able to make decisions for yourself. Studies have even shown that engaging in end-of-life care discussions and advanced care planning does not lead to an increased incidence of depression or anxiety. In fact, those who have end-of-life care discussions are more likely to accept the reality that their illness is terminal and will lead to death. This acceptance can lead to a more realistic and prepared mindset.

Relieving Family Burden:

Clearly documented preferences can relieve family members of the burden of making difficult decisions on your behalf, reducing potential conflicts and emotional stress. For those who have lost a loved one, there are improved bereavement outcomes when there have been open and honest discussions about end-of-life preferences. This can lead to a healthier grieving process. In essence, having these conversations is a proactive and positive step that helps individuals and families make informed decisions, ensure that care is aligned with personal values, and facilitate open communication during a challenging time.

Emotional and Spiritual Support during End-of-Life

Emotional and spiritual support is as important as physical treatment in most cases, and by having your emotional needs taken care of as part of a whole-person, holistic approach to your palliative care journey will ensure that you are able to enjoy a better quality of life until the very end.

As human beings, we are innately social creatures. We derive joy from the company of those we connect with on a deep emotional and intellectual level. And this truth holds steadfast even as we embark on our palliative care journey. There is no reason to believe that this beautiful aspect of our existence will change. Maybe you've always loved going to a weekly club or joining a society centered around a topic you enjoy. Or maybe you've taken weekend trips with a group that shares your interests. Or perhaps you simply like meeting up and chatting with a community group every week. Whatever it may be, there's absolutely no reason why you can't keep doing these things while going through palliative care. As long as you feel up to it, continue to embrace your passions and activities.

Sharing your feelings can also be incredibly helpful when navigating a stressful situation. So, consider reaching out to someone experienced in providing emotional support during your palliative care journey. There may be topics that are too difficult to discuss with loved ones, and that's where qualified counselors and therapists can truly make a positive impact on your final months and years. Trust in their expertise to make your journey a little easier.

Finally, if you've chosen to remain at home during your palliative care journey, then it's important to create a supportive atmosphere. Have friends and family come by for visits, and consider asking volunteers from your community group to help with housework or errands so that you don't feel overwhelmed. This can also be an opportunity to spend quality time with family and friends — something you may not otherwise do in your busy life. With the help of these supportive measures, you can make your journey easier and more enjoyable.

Now, spirituality, on the other hand, is a deeply personal experience. For some, it means being part of an established religion, going to services, and following specific practices and beliefs. For others, spirituality is more like their own belief system or philosophy of life on this planet and beyond.

As people approach the end of their lives, their perspectives on spirituality might change as they reflect on their existence and think about the meaning of life. This shift can make some individuals more aware of their spirituality, while others may experience spiritual anguish. When people start questioning their beliefs or get worried about the mismatch between their actions and spiritual beliefs, they go through spiritual distress. This might involve blaming God for their illness, asking for forgiveness for their wrongdoings, or feeling like their actions are beyond redemption.

Spiritual distress can have psychological and physical effects, impacting both the person and their loved ones. People with this kind of distress may have difficulty sleeping, become withdrawn, or even become suicidal. It's important to remember that spiritual distress can be treated. Hospice chaplains, counselors, and spiritual advisors can work with individuals to shape their beliefs and help them find peace again. Many people find solace in religious activities such as prayer or meditation, which can be a powerful restorative tool for those suffering from spiritual distress.

Patients receiving hospice or palliative care often have spiritual needs that encompass various aspects. These needs may involve connecting with their religious faith and practices, seeking understanding of what brings meaning to their life, exploring their desired legacy, seeking personal forgiveness, offering forgiveness to others, and sharing their life story. Hospice chaplains are there to actively listen to patients, addressing their spiritual inquiries and concerns. If requested, they can also help connect patients with spiritual leaders of their faith, like priests, rabbis, imams, or other ministers.

In the end, the goal of chaplains is for patients to reach a place of peace and comfort in their final days, providing support and understanding as they grapple with the struggles of mortality. This brings them comfort, solace, and a sense of peace as they transition from this life to the next.

Grief and Bereavement Support for Caregivers

As a caregiver, you may find yourself experiencing a variety of emotions over time. Some of the most profound emotions caregivers often encounter are feelings of loss and frustration. These emotions can be incredibly challenging to navigate, but there are strategies to cope with them. It is hard to see your loved one decline, and as a caregiver, you may be struggling with the moral and emotional challenges that come along with it. Grief is indeed a natural response to loss, and allowing yourself to experience the range of emotions that come with it is an essential part of healing.

As someone who has loved, cared for, lost, and finally grieved for a person with PD, I can tell you that you don't realize how much your life revolved around that person until they are gone. But there are other aspects of grief that I experienced that are common with severe illnesses and begin long before the person passes away.

Two types of loss that are common among caregivers are **ambiguous loss** and **anticipatory grief**. Ambiguous loss occurs when someone you care for is physically present but not the same person they used to be due to their condition. This can create a sense of loss even while the person is still alive. Anticipatory grief, on the other hand, arises when you are aware that a loss is imminent, and you begin to grieve before it actually happens.

In the early stages of caregiving, it's important to seek support and develop coping strategies for dealing with these emotions, even before you feel overwhelmed. Caregiving is not just about physical tasks; it also involves emotional and mental challenges. Many people may not fully comprehend the extent of the emotional and mental effort required if they have never had to do it.

In the late stages of Parkinson's disease, individuals will likely require assistance with most of their personal care needs. As the symptoms progress, they may struggle with walking and eventually lose the ability to stand. Non-movement symptoms such as hallucinations and delusions may also emerge. It's essential to collaborate closely with their medical team to explore ways to alleviate pain, enhance comfort, and provide quality care.

During this stage, caregivers become a vital link to ensuring quality care and services for the person with Parkinson's. Advocating for them and being their connection to care becomes even more critical when they can no longer advocate for themselves. There may come a point when the person requires a higher level of care than can be provided at home, necessitating a move to a nursing facility. While this decision can be emotionally challenging, it's essential to prioritize their safety and well-being. Even if the person with Parkinson's is moved to a skilled nursing facility, your role as a caregiver doesn't necessarily end. Your presence and advocacy are still vital to ensure proper care is administered.

Remember that caregiving can be demanding and emotionally taxing. Seeking help and support is not a sign of weakness but a necessary step to ensure your own well-being. By implementing healthy coping strategies, you can navigate the challenges of caregiving more effectively and maintain your own resiliency. In the end, after they are gone, you will have the satisfaction of knowing that you did your best to provide them with the support they needed.

Ultimately, it's important to be aware that there is no one-size-fits-all approach when it comes to caregiving for someone with Parkinson's disease. Everyone's situation is unique and each person requires a tailor-made approach that takes into account their individual circumstances and needs. That being said, there are healthy ways to manage feelings of anxiety, loss, and grief:

Feel Your Emotions: Embrace and allow yourself to experience the emotions that come with grief. Avoid suppressing or bottling up your feelings, as this can lead to prolonged and worsened emotional and physical health.

Take Care of Your Physical Health: Prioritize self-care, including getting enough sleep and maintaining a healthy diet. Grief can take a toll on your body, so taking care of your physical well-being is essential.

Stay Connected: Don't isolate yourself. Surround yourself with supportive friends, family, and loved ones who can provide care and understanding during the grieving process.

Engage in Positive Distractions: While it's important to process your emotions, engaging in activities you enjoy can provide healthy distractions and prevent you from dwelling on negative thoughts.

Reestablish Routines: Rebuilding your daily routines can help reduce stress, anxiety, and feelings of hopelessness. Gradually reintroduce structure into your life.

Understand Adaptation: Over time, you will adapt to the loss and experience fewer and less intense waves of grief. Grief is a process, and while it may feel overwhelming at first, you can adjust and find ways to cope.

And remember, you are not alone. Allow yourself to feel your emotions, and don't hesitate to reach out for support. With mindful self-care and empathy, you can heal from grief in time. In the end, it's not about losing hope or dwelling on the negative but rather about embracing the opportunity to have control over one's own care and creating a more peaceful and prepared journey for everyone involved.

Epilogue

"Everyone loves a story with a villain. It holds our attention and galvanizes us; it gives us a common enemy. In the field of neurodegenerative diseases, which include Parkinson's, Alzheimer's, and others, the victim is the brain, and the villain is the abnormal proteins." - Dr. Espay is the Endowed Chair of the James J. and Joan A. Gardner Center for Parkinson's disease at the University of Cincinnati

It is true when they say that PD is not something that happens to one person but to an entire family. Everyone is affected by the disease, and everyone needs help in coping with it. It is important to take advantage of every resource available when it comes to managing PD-related symptoms and improving the quality of life for both patients and caregivers.

For all the caregivers out there, as the caregiving role becomes more demanding, it's crucial to prioritize your own well-being and seek the support you need. Whether you're assisting your spouse or another loved one, remember that both their needs and your own matter. If you find yourself providing care in the middle of the night or experiencing burnout, it's okay to ask for help. There are resources available, friends and family who can offer assistance. Don't hesitate to lean on them and avoid carrying the burden alone.

Caregiving is a marathon, and it's important not to exhaust yourself along the way. As you adapt to changing circumstances, both taking care of your loved one and ensuring you're taking care of yourself are essential. As a caregiver for someone with this debilitating disease, I can attest to the fact that PD can be both emotionally and physically draining. However, it is even more devastating when you don't have the answers or the right resources to make sure your loved one is getting the best care possible. That is why I have tried my best to consolidate all the information I have gathered through my own research and from talking to other PD patients and caregivers. In this book, you can find the resources that I found most useful in managing the effects of Parkinson's disease on both patients and their families, from medication reminders to mobility aids. From support groups to mental health professionals, there is something for everyone when it comes to managing PD. I hope that by providing this information, I can help to make life a little easier for everyone affected by Parkinson's disease.

But this is not the end of the information. If you need to know more, there are tons of support groups and foundations that provide specialized advice and resources. Please take a few minutes to explore the websites of these organizations, as they offer invaluable insight into Parkinson's disease and its management.

1. Michael J. Fox Foundation for Parkinson's Research:

Founded in: 2000

Founder: Michael J. Fox

Overview: The Michael J. Fox Foundation for Parkinson's Research was established by actor Michael J. Fox, who was diagnosed with Parkinson's disease in 1991 at the age of 29. The foundation is dedicated to accelerating the development of improved treatments and, ultimately, a cure for Parkinson's disease. It funds research, promotes awareness, and advocates for policies that support the Parkinson's community. The foundation has played a significant role in advancing Parkinson's research and raising awareness about the disease. One of the more famous initiatives is Fox Trial Finder an online platform that connects individuals with clinical research opportunities related to Parkinson's disease. By signing up, you can join a community of people willing to participate in trials that could help researchers better understand the causes and treatments for Parkinson's disease.

2. Parkinson's Foundation:

Founded in 1957 (as the National Parkinson Foundation, later merged with Parkinson's Disease Foundation in 2016)

Overview: The Parkinson's Foundation, originally known as the National Parkinson Foundation, was established to support research and education related to Parkinson's disease. It merged with the Parkinson's Disease Foundation in 2016 to form a unified organization that provides resources, education, and advocacy for the Parkinson's community. One of the more famous research projects includes the Parkinson's Outcomes Project, which collects data on over 13,000 people with Parkinson's in order to better understand the impact of the disease. The foundation also provides support for people with Parkinson's, such as providing resources to help them better manage their symptoms and connect with others in the community. Additionally, they advocate for higher standards of care and improved access to treatments.

3. Davis Phinney Foundation:

Founded in: 2004

Founder: Davis Phinney, former professional cyclist

Overview: The Davis Phinney Foundation was founded by former professional cyclist Davis Phinney, who was diagnosed with young-onset Parkinson's disease. The foundation focuses on helping people with Parkinson's live well by promoting physical activity, wellness, and community engagement. It funds research projects and offers programs that aim to improve the quality of life for people living with Parkinson's.

4. National Parkinson Foundation (NPF):

Founded in: 1957

Overview: The National Parkinson Foundation was originally established to improve the care and quality of life for people with Parkinson's disease. It provides resources, support, and education for patients, caregivers, and healthcare professionals. The NPF also funds research initiatives and advocates for policies that benefit the Parkinson's community.

5. The Cure Parkinson's Trust:

Founded in: 2005

Overview: The Cure Parkinson's Trust was founded by four individuals with Parkinson's disease and their friends. This UK-based foundation focuses on funding research projects that aim to slow, stop, or reverse the progression of Parkinson's disease. The foundation aims to find ways to improve treatments and ultimately find a cure.

6. The Parkinson Alliance:

Founded in: 1999

Overview: The Parkinson Alliance is dedicated to raising funds for research to help find a cure for Parkinson's disease. It organizes various events and fundraising initiatives to support research projects aimed at advancing our understanding of Parkinson's and developing better treatments.

7. Brian Grant Foundation:

Founded in: 2010

Founder: Brian Grant, former NBA player

Overview: The Brian Grant Foundation was founded by former NBA player Brian Grant, who was diagnosed with Parkinson's disease in 2008. The foundation focuses on empowering individuals with Parkinson's to live active and fulfilling lives through exercise and wellness programs. It also supports research efforts to improve treatments and find a cure.

8. American Parkinson Disease Association (APDA):

Founded in: 1961

Overview: The American Parkinson Disease Association provides information, support, and resources for individuals and families affected by Parkinson's disease. The organization funds research projects, offers educational materials, and advocates for policies that improve the lives of people with Parkinson's.

9. European Parkinson's Disease Association (EPDA)/ Parkinson's Europe:

Founded in: 1992

Overview: The European Parkinson's Disease Association is a non-profit organization that works to improve the quality of life for people living with Parkinson's in Europe. Through advocacy, research funding, and patient support services, EPDA works to raise awareness and provide resources to individuals with Parkinson's and their families. They also work closely with policymakers and other stakeholders in order to ensure that their efforts are realized. EPDA also hosts educational events, organizes conferences, and provides information about clinical trials. Through their work, they strive to improve the quality of life for those affected by Parkinson's disease in Europe.

10. World Parkinson Coalition:

Founded in: 2006

Overview: The World Parkinson Coalition is a global nonprofit organization dedicated to improving the lives of people with Parkinson's disease. The WPC provides treatment, support, and advocacy for people with Parkinson's disease worldwide. They organize global conferences to discuss new developments in research and treatments, provide resources and education to those affected by Parkinson's disease, and promote awareness of the condition. They also work closely with healthcare providers, scientists, patients, caregivers, industry stakeholders, governments and policymakers to ensure that people impacted by Parkinson's disease get the best available treatment and support.

Each of these foundations has contributed significantly to advancing Parkinson's disease research, raising awareness, and supporting individuals and families affected by the condition. Through their efforts, people with Parkinson's can access resources to help them better manage the condition and live fulfilling lives. Together, these foundations form a network of support that continues to grow and make an impact.

A Request from The Author

"He who said money can't buy happiness, hasn't given enough away."

Unknown

Did you know that people who help others (with zero expectation) experience higher levels of fulfillment, live longer, and make more money? I'd like to create the opportunity to deliver this value to you during your reading or listening experience. To do so, I have a simple question for you...

Would you help someone you've never met if it didn't cost you money, but you never got credit for it?

If so, I have a favor to ask you to do on behalf of someone you do not know. And likely, never will.

The only way for us to accomplish our mission of helping patients with Parkinson's Disease and their caregivers is, first, by reaching them. And most people do, in fact, judge a book by its cover (and its reviews). If you have found this book valuable, would you please take a brief moment right now and leave an honest review of the book and its contents? It will cost you zero dollars and less than 60 seconds.

Your review will help...

one more patient to understand their diagnosis better.

one more caregiver to have the knowledge and tools to cope with the disease and its progression.

one more patient to understand the array of treatments and medication options that are available.

one more life to change for the better.

To make this happen...all you have to do is take less than 60 seconds and leave a review. –

Thank You!

About the Author

Rory Graham is a video producer and marketer with 39 years of experience and the owner of Allied Video Services. His passion is to find creative solutions to help his clients succeed in attracting, converting, and communicating with their prospects.

He is the creator and producer of "Hampton Roads Business Live" an online interview show that interviewed more than 400 local successful business owners in Hampton Roads.

Rory is the author of several books including "Did I Tell You I Love You Today?" and Finding Light in The Darkness."

He is a business speaker and trainer who has helped over 300 entrepreneurs in opening their own production companies across the United States.

Rory is very involved in community causes including the American Red Cross, Union Mission, the American Parkinson Disease Association, and others.

Rory has two sons and lives in Chesapeake, VA.

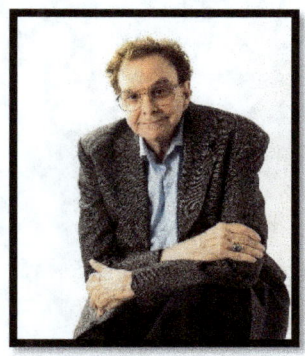